made **INCREDIBLY**

EASY!

Nursing Care Planning

Adapted for the UK by

Emily Matthews, RN, DipHE, BSc, MSc, PGCMedEd

Director of Professional Practice, Anglia Ruskin University

First UK Edition

Wolters Kluwer | Lippincott Williams & Wilkins
Health

Philadelphia · Baltimore · New York · London
Buenos Aires · Hong Kong · Sydney · Tokyo

Staff

Acquisitions Editor
Rachel Hendrick

Academic Marketing Executive
Alison Major

Production Editor
Kevin Johnson

Proofreader
Helena Engstrand

Illustrator
Bot Roda

Text and Cover Design
Designers Collective

Printed and bound by Euradius in the Netherlands
Typeset by MPS Limited, A Macmillan Company
For information, write to Lippincott Williams & Wilkins, 250 Waterloo Road, London SE1 8RD

British Library Cataloging-in-Publication Data. A catalogue record for this book is available from the British Library

ISBN-13: 978-1-901831-16-0
ISBN-10: 1-901831-16-7

Contents

Acknowledgements

Peterborough and Stamford Hospitals NHS Foundation Trust
Coronary Care Unit (Integrated Care Pathway)

Reviewers of the UK edition

Elizabeth Susan Clifton, SRN, NDN Cert, BSc, MSc, PGCE
Senior Lecturer in Adult Nursing, School of Health and Wellbeing, The University of Wolverhampton

Neal F Cook, BSc Hons, MSc, PG Dip, PG Cert, Dip Aromatherapy, IFPA, RN, Specialist Practitioner Adult, Lecturer/Practice Educator.
Lecturer in Nursing, University of Ulster

Cath Hill, PGD, PGCE BSC, RN
Lecturer, School of Nursing & Midwifery, Keele University

Alexandra Levine, MA, BSc(Hons), DipN(Lond), RN, Cert Ed
Senior Lecturer, Department of Nursing and Applied Clinical Studies, Faculty of Health and Social Care, Canterbury Christ Church University

Ian Stevenson, MA Ed (Merit), MSc, MA, BSc (Hons), BA, RGN, EN (G), RNMH, Diploma Management Studies (DMS), BTEC NVQ 5, ENB 806, CMH Cert, FETC, 730 C&G's, Cert Ed, RNT, FHEA, D32, D33, D34.
Senior Lecturer, Department of Nursing and Caring Sciences, University of Central Lancashire

Lynne Williams, MSc, BSc (Hons), RGN
Lecturer in Adult Nursing, School of Healthcare Sciences, Bangor University

Foreword to the UK edition

I am an advocate of the nursing process! Throughout my clinical and academic career, and indeed life in general, I have used the nursing process to help me make sense of situations and guide me in deciding what actions I should take. The nursing process has helped me to solve many problems, ranging from how best to care for my patients, to where I should go on holiday and in fact the nursing process is still my mantra for life. It is a process that works!

As a nurse in clinical practice, managing the delivery of patient care will require constant critical-thinking and problem-solving skills; however, developing these skills can be challenging. One tool for making critical thinking and problem solving less demanding is the nursing process; and one extraordinary resource for making the nursing process less unwieldy is *Care Planning Made Incredibly Easy.*

The nursing process is the foundation for professional nursing practice. It's the systematic, problem-solving method used to teach and guide nursing care planning. Practicing nurses use the nursing process as the framework for the clinical decision-making and critical thinking that are essential for safe, quality nursing practice. In addition, clinical guidelines, integrated care pathways and standardised care plans are all based on the nursing process.

Care Planning Made Incredibly Easy takes an innovative approach to nursing care planning in that it focuses on the skills necessary to develop patient-specific, relevant, timely nursing care plans. Divided into two sections, this newly adapted reference walks students step-by-step through the care planning process in a way that builds problem-solving and critical-thinking skills. Content that's particularly valuable to nursing students includes discussions about the differences between medical and nursing diagnoses; the relevance of nursing care planning to practice after graduation; the role of the nurse and nursing documentation in interdisciplinary care and the importance of evaluation throughout patient care. The importance of systematic problem-solving is emphasised throughout the text through the use of concept maps, sample case studies and sample care plan components. Important terms are defined and applied to aid student comprehension of these important concepts.

Part I of the book is dedicated to the development of a nursing care plan and details each step of the nursing process. Following the five-step nursing process—assessment, diagnosis, planning, implementation, and evaluation—each chapter includes a detailed discussion of the step and its application to nursing practice, with loads of practical application examples. Each chapter ends with *On the case*, a quiz that helps students hone their critical-thinking skills and gauge their comprehension of the content presented. Part II, 'Nursing diagnoses by medical diagnosis', is a handy resource that lists hundreds of examples of adult, maternal-neonatal, children's and mental health nursing diagnoses for the most common medical diagnoses.

Logos throughout the text make learning easy and focus the reader on essential information:

Under construction offers sample concept maps and care plan components, plus tips for making care plans patient-specific and individualised.

Weighing the evidence provides information on the latest evidenced-based standards of care used in the sample care plans.

Teacher knows best imparts important reminders that help students understand how to apply content.

Memory jogger mnemonic devices help students remember key concepts and content.

In summary, *Care Planning Made Incredibly Easy* is a valuable reference for nursing students learning the nursing process and nursing care planning. I believe this text will not only assist the student in learning how to develop an individualised care plan but, more importantly, it will provide a framework for using the nursing process to better understand the clinical presentation and nursing care needs of the patient as well as to promote systematic problem-solving and clinical judgement.

Emily Matthews
RN, DipHE, BSc, MSc, PGCMedEd
Director of Professional Practice
Faculty of Health and Social Care
Anglia Ruskin University

Advisory board to the US edition

Contributors and consultants to the US edition

Melody C. Antoon, RN, MSN
Instructor
Lamar State College
Port Arthur, TX

Elizabeth (Libby) A. Archer, RN, EDD
Associate Professor
Baptist College of Health Sciences
Memphis, TN

Peggy D. Baikie, RNC, MS, NNP, PNP
Clinical Coordinator/Nurse Practitioner
St. Anthony Hospitals

Denver
Adjunct Professor
Metropolitan State College of Denver

Mary Elaine Bell-Braxton, RN, MS
Adjunct Faculty & Nursing Resource
Center Coordinator
University of West Georgia
Carrollton, GA

Cheryl L. Brady, RN, MSN
Assistant Professor
Kent State University
Salem, OH

Stephanie C. Butkus, RN, MSN, CPNP, IBCLC
Assistant Professor, Division of Nursing
Kettering (Ohio) College of Medical Arts

Joanna E. Cain, RN, BSN
President
Auctorial Pursuits, Inc.
Wilmington, NC

Julie Calvery, RN, MS
Instructor
University of Arkansas, Fort Smith, AR

Cynthia A. Chatham, RNC, DSN
Associate Professor
University of Southern Mississippi School
of Nursing
Long Beach, MS

Wendy Tagan Conroy, MSN, FNP, BC
Advanced Practice Registered Nurse
Connecticut Valley Hospital
Middletown, CT

Charlotte Conway, RN, MSN
Per Diem Staff Nurse, Pediatric
Intensive Care
Santa Clara Valley Medical Center
San Jose, CA

Linda Carman Copel, RN, PhD, CGP, CS, DAPA
Associate Professor
Villanova (PA) University

Linda Crawford, RN, MSN
Assistant Professor of Practical Nursing
Coastal Georgia Community College
Brunswick, GA

Kim R. Davis, RN, MSN
Nurse Manager, MICU and SICU
Ralph H. Johnson VA Medical Center
Charleston, SC

Valerie J. Flattes, APRN, BC-ANP
Clinical Instructor
University of Utah College of Nursing
Salt Lake City, UT

Erica Fooshee, RN, MSN
Nursing Instructor
Department of Nursing
Pensacola (FL) Junior College

Candace Furlong, APRN, BC, MSN, CNS, NP
Professor, Nursing
American River College
Sacramento, CA

Rhonda Gall, APRN, BC, GNP
Lecturer
Bowie (MD) State University

Janis Guilbeau, RN, MSN
Instructor of Nursing
University of Louisiana
Lafayette, LA

Kenneth Hazell, ARNP, MSN, PhD(C)
Nursing Program Director
Keiser University
Ft. Lauderdale, FL

Connie S. Heflin, RN, MSN
Professor
West Kentucky Community
and Technical College
Paducah, KY

Julia Anne Isen, RN, MS, FNP-C
Assistant Clinical Professor, School
of Nursing
University of California
San Francisco, CA

Karla Jones, RN, MN
Nursing Department Faculty
Treasure Valley Community College
Ontario, OR

Rebecca Frey Keller, ARNP, MSN
Nursing Instructor
Keiser College
Fort Lauderdale, FL

Merita Konstantacos, RN, MSN
Consultant
Clinton, OH

Cheryl Laskowski, APRN-BC, DNS
Assistant Professor of Nursing
University of Vermont
Burlington;
Advanced Practice Nurse
Center for Pain Medicine
South Burlington, VT

Rosemary Macy, RN, PhD
Associate Professor
Boise (Idaho) State University

Judith A. Murphy, RN, BSN
Ambulatory Nurse
Cambridge Health Alliance
Medford, MA

Noel C. Piano, RN, MS
Instructor/Coordinator
Lafayette School of Practical Nursing
Adjunct Faculty;
Thomas Nelson Community College
Williamsburg, VA

Melody F. Pope, RN, MSED, MSN
Assistant Professor of Nursing
College of the Redwoods
Crescent City, CA

Monica Narvaez Ramirez, RN, MSN
Nursing Instructor
University of the Incarnate Word School of
Nursing & Health Professions
San Antonio, TX

Debra L. Renna, CCRN, MSN
Professor of Nursing
Keiser College
Fort Lauderdale, FL

Nan C. Riedè, RN, MSN
Assistant Professor
Baptist College of Health Sciences
Memphis, TN

Barbara K. Scheirer, RN, MSN
Assistant Professor
School of Nursing
Grambling (LA) State University

Kendra S. Seiler, RN, MSN
Nursing Instructor
Rio Hondo College
Whittier, CA

Georgia Simmons, RN, BSN
Practical Nursing Instructor
Ivy Tech Community College
Madison, IN

Sheryl Thomas, RN, MSN
Nurse Instructor
Wayne County Community College
Detroit, MI

Phyllis Tipton, RN, PhD
ADN Instructor
McLennan Community College
Research Coordinator
Hillcrest Baptist Medical Center
Waco, TX

Kathleen Tusaie, APRN, BC, PhD
Assistant Professor/Advanced
Practice Nurse
The University of Akron (OH) College
of Nursing

Patricia Van Tine, RN, MA, CPT
Nursing Educator
Mt. San Jacinto College
Menifee, CA

Ralph Vogel, RN, PhD, CPNP
Assistant Clinical Professor
College of Nursing
University of Arkansas for
Medical Sciences
Little Rock, AR

**Sandra K. Voll, RNC, MS, CNM,
FNP, WHNP**
Clinical Assistant Professor, Director of
Clinical Learning Center
Virginia Commonwealth University School
of Nursing
Richmond, VA

Kelly Witter, RN, MSN, CLC
Director, Practical Nursing Program
Great Oaks Career Campuses
Cincinnati, OH

Hollace Yowler, RN, MSN
Associate Professor
Ivy Tech Community College
Madison, IN

Part I

Care planning using the nursing process

① Introduction to care planning

Just the facts

In this chapter, you'll learn:

♦ the benefits of using the nursing process

♦ the role of the nursing process in planning patient-centred care

♦ ways in which the nursing process promotes critical thinking

♦ fundamentals of concept mapping and its uses in care planning.

A look at care planning

A crucial component of nursing care, a care plan (also known as a *plan of care*) serves as a road map that guides all staff members involved in a patient's care. Care planning allows a nurse to identify a patient's problems and select interventions that will help solve or minimise these problems.

The great communicator

The care plan also communicates vital patient information to the entire health care team. It contains detailed instructions for achieving the goals established for the patient.

Understanding the nursing process

Effective care planning results from the nursing process—a deliberate, systematic process that takes a problem-solving approach to nursing care. Development and acceptance of the nursing process is one of the key advances in nursing over the past few decades.

> Think of a care plan as a map that helps the health care team stay on course when it comes to patient care.

Analyse, address, implement, evaluate

The cornerstone of nursing, the nursing process, gives you a structure for applying your knowledge and skills in an organised, goal-orientated way. It helps you think critically, solve problems and make care decisions tailored to each patient's individual needs.

The nursing process requires you to systematically analyse patient data, make inferences, draw conclusions about patient problems and devise a care plan to address those problems, implement the plan, evaluate the plan's effectiveness and revise the plan if necessary.

Oh, the humanity

The nursing process is holistic and humanistic. It addresses the human response to medical conditions—how these conditions affect the patient's life. To use it correctly, you must consider not just the individual's physical, mental and emotional status, but also their interests, values, beliefs, and ethnic, religious and cultural background.

Advantages of the nursing process

When used effectively, the nursing process offers many advantages:
- It's patient-centred, helping to ensure that your patient's health problems and his response to them are the focus of care.
- It enables you to individualise care for each patient.
- It promotes the patient's participation in their care, encourages independence and concordance and gives the patient a greater sense of control—important factors in a positive health outcome. (See *Putting the 'P' in planning*.)
- It improves communication by providing you and other nurses with a summary of the patient's recognised problems or needs.

Teacher knows best

Putting the 'P' in planning

Always remember to include the 'P'—the patient—in planning. Ask for your patient's input when identifying his problems, establishing outcomes and formulating interventions. Doing this validates their importance as an individual and motivates them to participate in their health care and adhere to the care plan. It also gives them a greater sense of control, which promotes personal responsibility and strengthens their commitment to working toward the established goals.

- It promotes accountability for nursing activities, which in turn promotes quality assurance.
- It promotes critical thinking, decision-making and problem-solving.
- It's outcome-focused and encourages the evaluation of results.
- It minimises errors and omissions in care planning.

Basis for the nursing process

The nursing process is based on the scientific method of problem-solving, which involves:
- stating the problem you observed
- forming a hypothesis about the solution to the problem ('if . . . then' statements)
- developing a method to test the hypothesis
- collecting the test data
- analysing the data
- drawing conclusions about the hypothesis.

> Picking out shoes is scientific? I knew there was a good reason it took me so long—I just always thought it was all of the shoes.

A scientific fact

Most people use the scientific method instinctively, without being aware they're doing it. Simply picking out which pair of shoes best complements your favourite outfit is an exercise in the scientific method. So if you're familiar with the scientific process, the nursing process probably seems familiar.

Nursing process steps

The nursing process encompasses five steps:

 assessment

nursing diagnosis

 planning

implementation

 evaluation.

Following these steps systematically in this order enables you to organise and prioritise patient care—especially critical for the novice nursing student. It also helps ensure that you don't skip or overlook important information. (See *Just how many steps are there?*, page 6.)

When used correctly, the nursing process ensures that the care plan is revised when new problems arise or patient outcomes remain unmet. It also allows the care plan to be discontinued when patient outcomes have been met.

Just how many steps are there?

Nurses are accountable for all aspects of their practice, including the way in which they use the nursing process to organise and deliver nursing care (NMC 2008). However, the number of stages in the nursing process is something that is hotly debated!

The initial definition of the nursing process from the 1950s listed only three steps: assessment, planning and evaluation; however, depending on who you ask, the nursing process can now consist of four, five or even six stages:

- assessment
- nursing diagnosis
- outcome identification
- planning
- implementation
- evaluation.

In the United Kingdom, the nursing process has traditionally been seen as consisting of four steps—assess, plan, implement and evaluate—with nursing diagnosis incorporated into the assessment stage and outcome identification forming the first part of the planning stage.

In this book, we are going to continue to focus on a five-step process that includes nursing diagnosis as a separate stage between assessment and planning, as this provides the most effective framework for getting to grips with the nursing process.

Remember that the nursing process guides all the nurse's *actions* and *decisions,* regardless of the number of steps cited.

Domino effect

Although the five nursing process steps are sequential, they are also continuous and overlapping. For instance, when performing an intervention, such as changing your patient's dressing, you should also be assessing his skin. (See *The nursing process: An unbroken circle*.)

What's more, these steps are inter-related, with each one influencing all the subsequent steps. For instance:
- Your assessment must be thorough and accurate so that you formulate the appropriate nursing diagnosis.
- The nursing diagnosis you formulate must be appropriate to ensure that you choose reasonable outcomes.
- The outcomes you identify must be appropriate so that you outline correct interventions.
- The interventions you choose must be appropriate so that your patient will make progress toward the outcomes you've established.

The nursing process: An unbroken circle

The nursing process is a progression of actions that continually recycle as patient problems and priorities change or resolve. In any specific task you do, more than one step may be involved.

Take for example …

When you initially assess a new patient's ability to meet their own hygiene needs, you begin the process of determining if the patient has any actual or potential problems related to washing and dressing. When you have diagnosed any problems you would then plan the interventions that enable the patient's personal hygiene needs to be met and as you implement the interventions planned in relation to personal hygiene you would assess the skin integrity on the patient's pressure areas.

The next time you support the patient with washing and dressing, you evaluate whether the interventions were effective in enabling the patient to meet their hygiene needs. However, if when you did this, you noticed that the skin on the patient's sacrum was becoming red—a change from your initial *assessment*—you would:

- conclude that the patient has been able to wash and dress with the support given (*evaluation*)
- identify that the patient is now at risk for pressure ulcer development (*nursing diagnosis*)
- identify that the patient's skin should be prevented from deteriorating further and should return to normal (*planning expected outcomes*)
- determine that you should ask the patient how he's feeling to identify associated symptoms, carry out a detailed pressure ulcer risk assessment to identify what equipment should be used, or actions taken, to prevent further breakdown, document this change in the patients skin integrity and notify the nurse in charge of the change (*planning interventions*)
- put your devised plan into action (*implementation*).

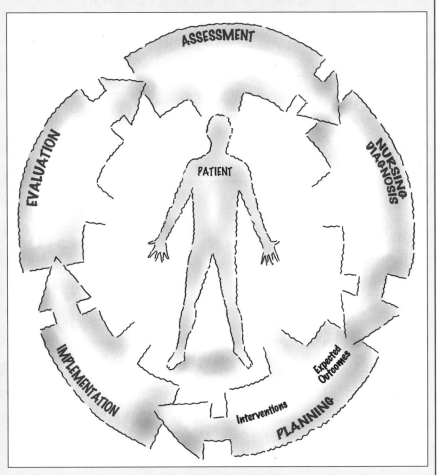

Under construction

Actual vs. At Risk of nursing diagnoses

When formulating your patient's nursing diagnoses, you need to specify whether your patient has each problem or is at risk of developing it. Here's the distinction:

- If the patient has identifiable signs and symptoms that appear in all or most patients with the disorder, you should label the problem with an *actual* nursing diagnosis.
- If the patient has risk factors for a problem but doesn't have signs or symptoms, you should label the problem with a *Risk of* diagnosis. This can also be referred to as a *potential* problem.

Take impaired skin integrity, for example. If the patient has erythema or an open skin area, they have *actual* impaired skin integrity and their diagnosis would be *Impaired skin integrity.* If they have no signs of skin breakdown but are bed-bound and have bowel and bladder incontinence, they have predisposing factors that place them at risk for impaired skin integrity; therefore, their nursing diagnosis would be *Risk of impaired skin integrity.*

If you go astray during any step—say, by misinterpreting the assessment data—you can get back on track by reassessing the patient, evaluating his care plan and revising the plan if necessary.

Assessment

The first step in the nursing process, assessment, involves the systematic collection of patient data. A comprehensive assessment gives you a wide-angle view of your patient's health problems, aiding in crucial decisions about patient care.

Nursing diagnosis

The second step requires you to use your assessment data to identify the patients problems or needs and formulate nursing diagnoses—clinical judgments about the patient's response to an actual or potential health problem that relate to the care that nurses deliver. (See *Actual vs. At Risk of nursing diagnoses.*) Remember, nursing diagnoses are different from medical diagnoses. (See *How nursing and medical diagnoses differ.*)

After the patient's problems or responses have been identified and reframed as nursing diagnoses, a quick review of the assessment findings and diagnoses can help you to correctly prioritise the most urgent needs of the patient.

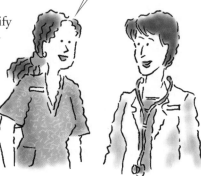

Although both are important parts of patient care, medical and nursing diagnoses are different.

How nursing and medical diagnoses differ

Medical practitioners (doctors) usually diagnose and treat medical conditions related to anatomy, physiology, disease or trauma. They formulate medical diagnoses that centre on these medical diseases and conditions.

The diagnosis of medical diseases and conditions is not part of most nurses' role. Instead, they formulate nursing diagnoses that focus on how the patient responds to the medical disease or condition. Unlike medical diagnoses, nursing diagnoses are patient-centred, and a nursing diagnosis may also help inform the medical diagnosis.

This case study will help you understand the difference between medical and nursing diagnoses.

Point, counterpoint

Mr Mills is a 52-year-old man who was hospitalised after falling on a patch of ice and injuring his right hip. He's married and has two children, one of whom attends University. Mr Mills works as a construction foreman; his wife is unemployed.

The practitioner's viewpoint

Here's how the doctor sees the situation: Mr Mills presents with pain in the right hip, a shortened right leg and external rotation of the right hip after sustaining a fall on a patch of ice. The hip x-ray shows a well-defined intertrochanteric fracture of the right hip. The medical diagnosis is a *right hip fracture*. The medical plan is to proceed with open reduction and internal fixation of the hip.

The nurse's perspective

Here's how the nurse views the same patient information: Mr Mills has pain in his right hip. He expresses an immediate concern about the need to urinate. He's also concerned about his job and lack of income during the recuperation period, when he won't be able to work. He says he has always been the breadwinner of his family, and he's worried that if he needs to be off work for a long time, he won't have the money to pay his son's university fees. The initial nursing diagnoses for Mr Mills are *Acute pain related to right hip fracture; Impaired urinary elimination related to inability to stand, pain and voluntary retention; Anxiety related to financial concerns and Anxiety related to anticipated loss of roles as employee and family provider.*

The differences

The nurse focuses on Mr Mills and his *responses* to the hip fracture. She isn't able to make independent decisions about how to treat the patient's hip fracture but can address the problems stemming from his responses to the fracture, such as pain and discomfort, concern with urination and the expected role change.

The nursing care plan should address Mr Mills' pain management needs, should include education about the indwelling urinary catheter that the nurse will place, a social worker referral to address Mr Mills' financial concerns and assistance in working through his expected role changes.

Three's company

Each nursing diagnosis has three components:
- label—an actual or potential problem that nursing care can affect
- related factors—factors that may precede, contribute to or be associated with the human response
- evidence—signs and symptoms that point to the nursing diagnosis.

Suppose, for instance, that your patient has constipation resulting from use of opioid analgesics for pain. You would formulate a nursing diagnosis of *Constipation related to use of opioid analgesics as evidenced by passage of hard, formed stools.*

One thing leads to another

Correctly identifying the problem and its cause is crucial to the next steps of the nursing process—planning and implementation.

Planning

During the planning stage of the nursing process, you:
- identify expected patient outcomes, or goals
- select nursing interventions designed to achieve these outcomes
- document the care plan, which becomes a permanent part of the patient's record and communicates the patient's needs to all health care practitioners who use the plan.

Here come the outcomes

For every nursing diagnosis, you must identify expected 'SMART' outcomes—specific, measurable, achievable, realistic and time-specific outcomes the patient should reach as a result of the nursing interventions you've planned. These outcomes are sometimes referred to as 'goals' or 'objectives'.

Outcomes derive from the nursing diagnosis. You must state them in terms of the patient's behaviour. For example, if the patient has a nursing diagnosis of *Lack of knowledge related to care of surgical wound*, one reasonable outcome might be 'Patient will describe precautions to take to prevent infection before discharge home.'

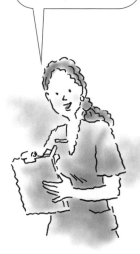

Don't forget documentation. It's an important part of the process.

Next in line—the interventions

Once you've identified the patient's problem or response and determined a reasonable outcome measurement, you can begin to list the steps that must be taken to reach that goal. Interventions are brief descriptions of specific actions. They should be based on the best evidence and they should conform to appropriate standards of care.

Don't forget to document

Always document the care plan so it's accessible to other staff members. Doing this provides crucial patient information to other health care team members, promoting continuity of care. Remember if you are a student nurse all of your entries in patient's documentation must be counter-signed by your mentor or another registered nurse.

Implementation

The next step in the nursing process is implementation, when you perform the actual interventions to help your patient reach the expected outcomes. But before carrying out these interventions, be sure to quickly reassess the patient to make sure that the interventions you've planned are still necessary. Patient situations can change rapidly, making some interventions inappropriate or unnecessary.

Throughout your nursing care, you'll need to evaluate the effectiveness of your interventions and make changes as needed. If you continue to implement ineffective interventions, you and your patient will lose valuable time. (See *Be flexible about care plans*.)

Evaluation

During the evaluation step of the nursing process, you:
- reassess the patient
- compare your findings with the outcome criteria or goals you established during the planning step
- determine the extent of outcome achievement—whether the goal was fully met, partially met or not met at all
- write evaluation statements
- revise the care plan as needed.

Although technically the last step of the nursing process, evaluation is an ongoing process that occurs each time you see the patient. You must continually evaluate the patient's response to interventions. (See *The focus factor*, page 12.)

A change of plans

If desired outcomes have been achieved, then this problem or need can be discontinued. If an outcome has been partially met, the plan may be continued with an extended time line.

If a desired outcome hasn't been met, you must re-examine the care plan and make necessary changes. To change the plan, you may need to review the new assessment data, formulate new diagnoses, establish new outcomes and select new interventions. Then update the written care plan accordingly. If the outcome has been met then the care plan may be discontinued.

How the nursing process promotes critical thinking

To use the nursing process, you must be able to think critically. Critical thinking is a disciplined mental process of analysing problems or phenomena that have been gathered from observation, experience, reflection, reasoning or communication.

Teacher knows best

Be flexible about care plans

The nursing care plan isn't set in stone. It must be updated as your patient's problems, needs and priorities change. Be sure to review the care plan often and modify it when necessary.

Teacher knows best

The focus factor

Stay focused during all interactions with your patient. To do this, you'll need to use active listening skills and turn off other thoughts going through your head, including 'What should I make for dinner?' and 'What time is my dentist appointment tomorrow?' Most patients are aware of the amount of focus and interest you bring to an exchange and will respond in kind.

Deliberate, purposeful and conscious, critical thinking requires reasonable, rational interpretation and evaluation of information. It leads you to reasonable solutions to a problem and helps you choose among these possible solutions to make a decision.

Hallmarks of critical thinking
The hallmarks of critical thinking are:
- clear, careful and precise thinking
- objective analysis of the evidence
- use of logical reasoning to reach a discriminating decision
- elimination of stereotypical thinking, bias, preconceptions and emotionally charged thinking.

A model process
The nursing process is a model of critical thinking because each step is purposeful, deliberate and designed to attain a certain goal. (See *Critical thinking: An essential skill.*)

For instance, when evaluating the assessment data you've gathered, you must think critically to determine which questions to ask your patient next. If he says he occasionally experiences chest pain, the critically thinking nurse doesn't simply record this statement and move on to the next topic. Instead, she asks questions designed to elicit details about the chest pain, such as:
- When does the pain occur? Do you experience it after strenuous physical activity? Does it occur after meals? While resting?
- How severe is the pain on a scale of 0 to 10?
- Do you have other problems along with the pain?
- Does the pain radiate to other parts of your body?

Risky factors
Thinking critically during assessment enables you to recognise factors that place your patient at increased risk of developing a problem. If you detect such a potential, you'll know the care plan should include a *Risk of* nursing diagnosis and appropriate interventions to prevent the problem.

Critical thinking: An essential skill

In the complex, rapidly changing health care environment, safe and effective nursing care demands critical thinking. Taking basic problem solving one step further, critical thinking considers all related factors, including the patient's unique needs and individual differences. Critical-thinking skills allow the nurse to step outside the situation and look at the whole picture more objectively.

Truth seekers

To obtain this complete picture, critical thinkers seek the truth and actively pursue answers to questions. They're also open-minded and creative and can draw from past clinical experiences to come up with all possible alternatives and then zero in on the best solution for the patient.

Practice for your practice

Books, articles and online courses are available to help nurses develop critical-thinking skills. Critical-thinking skills also develop as you reflect on your experiences and learn from them. When nurses engage in critical thinking, their patients have the best chances for success.

Likewise, critical thinking helps you write outcomes in a way that promotes easier evaluation and makes the need for any revisions readily apparent.

Novices need it, too

Critical thinking skills are essential for nurses at every level. As a newly qualified, novice nurse, you'll encounter situations you didn't see or learn about during your training—complex problems that require sound decision-making skills. You'll be expected to make important patient-care decisions and take actions based on those decisions.

As technology grows more advanced, such decisions and actions are becoming increasingly complex. What's more, they require you to analyse many patient variables, including social, cultural, emotional, physical, financial and spiritual issues.

Using the nursing process after qualification and registration

No matter how well you are supported in your first nursing job, you'll confront many new and unfamiliar situations and this will continue throughout your career. You'll need to make many on-the-spot decisions—some of which will be crucial. Using the nursing process and critical-thinking skills will help you succeed no matter what your responsibilities are. As you become more familiar with the nursing process, gain experience writing care plans and enhance

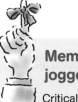

Memory jogger

Critical thinking is a life skill as well as a nursing essential. To remember the characteristics of critical-type thought, think of **CLOUD**:

Clear

Logical

Objective

Unbiased

Dispassionate (not emotion-driven).

your critical-thinking skills, your clinical judgment and ability to make good decisions will undoubtedly improve as your expertise develops.

Roll with the changes

Because the patient's status is dynamic and can change quickly, the nursing process is dynamic as well. As your patient's condition changes, you must assess these changes quickly and adjust the care plan appropriately. Use the nursing process as a road map and critical thinking as the vehicle to take you and your patient to the destination—the desired patient outcome.

Rinse and repeat

As you gain experience, you'll see that the nursing process shows you when and how to stop a nursing intervention—namely, when the desired outcomes are met. Or, if the outcomes remain unmet, the nursing process will lead you to reassess the situation and, if necessary, repeat the entire process.

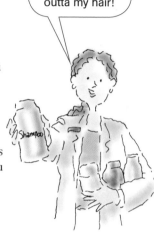

I'm gonna wash that diagnosis right outta my hair!

Concept mapping

A common tool to assist you in critical thinking is a concept map (sometimes called a *mind map* or *spider diagram*). A concept map is a diagram that shows relationships among various concepts. Concept mapping is a tool for visualising how concepts relate to one another. It helps you understand your patient's problems and care needs—and see how these items interact with each other.

A concept map helps you organise your thinking and see the big clinical picture. Each concept is enclosed in a box or circle, with lines between related concepts. Concept maps are especially helpful if you're a visual learner.

Comparing concept mapping and care planning

Concept mapping and traditional nursing care planning both have a problem-solving focus. However, concept mapping doesn't require linear design, which can hinder the free flow of ideas. It lets you view information in different ways and from different viewpoints because concepts aren't locked into specific positions. (See *Quick comparison*.)

Advantages of concept mapping

Concept mapping also has these other advantages over the traditional care plan:
• It makes the seemingly intangible concepts of patient problems, causes and effects more manageable.
• It clearly defines the central concept (the patient problem) by positioning it in the centre of the page. This ensures that the patient—not the medical diagnosis—is the focus.

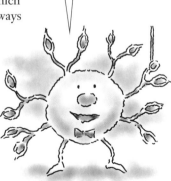

Concept mapping is similar to the brain's neural network. Each concept has long fibres that reach out and connect to other concepts.

Quick comparison

Here's a quick comparison of concept mapping and nursing care plans.

Concept map	Nursing care plan
• Visually organised	• Linearly organised
• Assessment data clearly linked to nursing problems (diagnoses)	• Assessment data usually in separate area or different form
• Good for quick identification and outline of multiple patient problems	• Good for quick communication of priority problems, outcomes and interventions

- It shows the relative importance of each concept.
- It helps you identify relationships between important concepts.
- It requires much less time to write than a care plan.
- It encourages creative and innovative ideas.
- It provides all the basic information on one page.
- It allows new information to be easily added.
- It enables you to see contradictions and gaps in the material or its interpretation, which provides a foundation for questioning, discovery and creativity.

Disadvantages of concept mapping

Despite its advantages, concept mapping can have certain drawbacks:
- Getting the map just right can be time consuming. You may have to redraw it several times until you're satisfied.
- It may become complex and cluttered, hindering your ability to see the big picture.
- It doesn't easily lend itself to standardised formats for everyday use in the clinical setting.

Nevertheless, concept mapping is a good way to develop the skills necessary to be able to effectively use the nursing process for care planning and is particularly helpful for students who are developing their knowledge and skills. These skills can then be adapted to the varying formats for care planning that you will encounter in clinical placements.

Creating a concept map

To develop a concept map for your patient, start with a clean sheet of unlined paper. (If you must use lined paper, turn it so the lines are vertical.) Then follow these steps:
- After you've assessed your patient, place a circle representing the patient in the middle of the paper. In this circle, write the patient's name or initials, chief complaint and medical diagnosis. By placing the patient in the centre of the page, your focus is clearly patient-centred. Remember, be brief!

- Write the patient's major problems or nursing diagnoses in boxes surrounding the patient, along with pertinent supporting data.
- Use lines to connect the central circle—the patient—to the nursing diagnoses boxes. You may also draw lines between related nursing diagnoses. For example, for a postoperative patient experiencing constipation caused by use of opioid analgesics, you would draw a line between the nursing diagnoses of *Acute pain* and *Constipation* to show that you understand they're related.
- Write expected outcomes for each nursing diagnosis; place each outcome in its own box because corresponding interventions will differ for each outcome. Connect these boxes with lines to the appropriate nursing diagnosis.
- In the same way, write interventions in a box for each outcome, followed by evaluations. Draw lines between each part of the nursing process to link related concepts. (See *Concept mapping without tears*.)

Patterns, symbols and notes

To help clarify your concept map, try using patterns and symbols to help organise types of information, such as:
- branches, to show how a concept can branch into ideas that are either closely or distantly related
- arrows, to join ideas from different branches
- circled groupings, to combine several branches of related ideas.
  You may also include explanatory notes—such as a few words, phrases or sentences—to explain, question or comment on a particular point.

Teacher knows best

Concept mapping without tears

These guidelines can help you to learn how to quickly and easily create concept maps:

- Work quickly without pausing. Try to keep up with the flow of ideas. Don't stop to decide where something should go or to organise the material. Just get it down on paper. Ordering and analysing are linear activities that can disrupt the mapping process.
- Write down everything you can think of without judging or editing—these activities can also disrupt the flow of concept mapping.
- If you come to a standstill, look over what you've done to see if you've left anything out.
- Confine the map to one page so it's easier to use.
- Print in capital letters for greater legibility. This also encourages you to keep the points brief.
- Initially, you may want to use colour coding to group sections of the map. As you gain experience, you'll probably find that colour coding isn't necessary.

Using your concept map

Concept maps are such useful tools that they can be used for multiple purposes. For example, you can use a concept map to explore a case study that you are using for one of your assignments or to guide your patient care during clinical placements. During your placements, you can carry your concept map in your pocket or place it in your clinical assessment booklet so you can refer to it often and update or revise it as necessary. But remember that when you write down any information about a patient, you have a duty to maintain their confidentiality and must protect their privacy in accordance with the Nursing and Midwifery Council Code of Conduct (NMC, 2008).

On the case

Case study background

Mr Jones is a 58-year-old male who was admitted to the acute admissions unit with cholecystitis. The patient reports pain in his abdomen, nausea and vomiting. His vital signs are as follows: heart rate 102 beats/minute, blood pressure 142/88 mmHg, oral temperature 38.2°C and respiratory rate 22 breaths/minute.

The patient rates his pain as an 8 on a scale of 0 to 10, with 10 being the most severe pain possible and 0 being the absence of pain. A nasogastric (NG) tube has been inserted and an intravenous line with dextrose 5% in normal saline solution has been started at 125 ml/hour. Mr Jones is scheduled for a laparoscopic cholecystectomy tomorrow.

Concept mapping exercise

Follow the steps outlined here to create a rough concept map for the care of Mr Jones. Don't worry if you can't complete the entire care plan. This is just your first try. The answers can be found at the end of this chapter.

Steps

1. Assess the patient to collect relevant information.
2. Write the patient's name or initials, medical diagnosis and chief complaint in the middle of a sheet of paper.
3. Write appropriate nursing diagnoses in boxes around the central box that contains the patient's name or initials and chief complaint. (*Hint:* One of the diagnoses should be *Acute pain.*)
4. Categorise assessment data under the appropriate nursing diagnoses.
5. Analyse the relationships among nursing diagnoses and draw lines to indicate these relationships.
6. On another piece of paper, identify patient goals, expected outcomes and nursing interventions for the nursing diagnosis *Acute pain*. Or, instead of using another piece of paper, you can create additional boxes on your

concept map for the goals, outcomes and interventions and then link these boxes to the related nursing diagnoses.

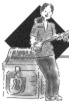

Answer key

Concept mapping exercise

Steps 1, 2, 3, 4 and 5
This concept map is one example of many possibilities for this patient. If you couldn't complete this concept map, don't worry. The remaining chapters in this book will walk you step-by-step through the process of creating a concept map that incorporates each stage of the nursing process.

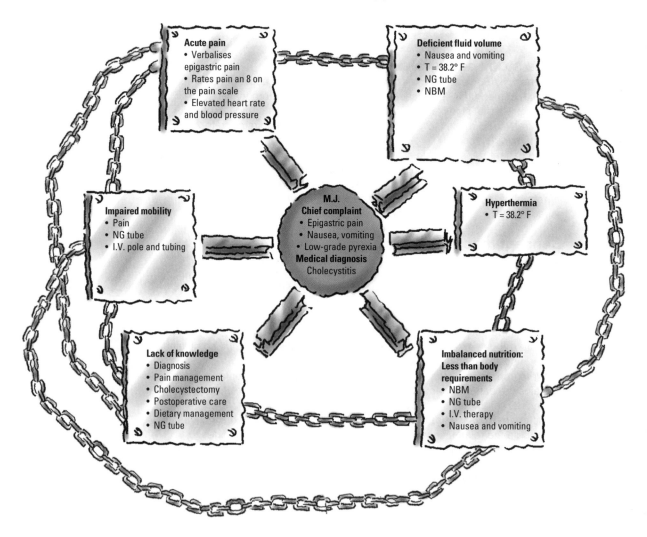

Acute pain
• Verbalises epigastric pain
• Rates pain an 8 on the pain scale
• Elevated heart rate and blood pressure

Deficient fluid volume
• Nausea and vomiting
• T = 38.2° F
• NG tube
• NBM

Impaired mobility
• Pain
• NG tube
• I.V. pole and tubing

M.J.
Chief complaint
• Epigastric pain
• Nausea, vomiting
• Low-grade pyrexia
Medical diagnosis
Cholecystitis

Hyperthermia
• T = 38.2° F

Lack of knowledge
• Diagnosis
• Pain management
• Cholecystectomy
• Postoperative care
• Dietary management
• NG tube

Imbalanced nutrition:
Less than body
requirements
• NBM
• NG tube
• I.V. therapy
• Nausea and vomiting

Step 6

Here's an example of a goal, expected outcomes and nursing interventions for the nursing diagnosis *Acute pain*:

• *Nursing diagnosis:* acute pain related to inflammation of the gallbladder as evidenced by the patient reporting pain rating as an 8 on a 0-to-10 scale— *Nursing priority:* pain control

• *Expected outcome:* patient's self-reported pain level is reduced to 3 on a 0-to-10 scale within 1 hour of initiation of prescribed analgesics.

Nursing interventions	Evaluation
Assess pain using pain scale.	*This section will include the patient's responses to the interventions on the left.*
Administer prescribed analgesia as appropriate.	
Instruct patient on use of patient-controlled analgesia, if appropriate.	
Assist the patient in to a comfortable position.	
Use techniques of relaxation, meditation or guided imagery.	

② Assessment

Just the facts

In this chapter, you'll learn:

♦ the components of a complete health assessment

♦ techniques and formats for gathering and organising assessment data

♦ tips for reviewing a patient's documentation for assessment data

♦ the steps for creating a concept map using assessment information.

A look at assessment

The first step in the nursing process, assessment, involves data collection to identify the patient's actual and potential health problems and needs. The goal is to gather as much information about your patient as possible. Using this data, you'll identify their needs, formulate nursing diagnoses, establish expected outcomes and identify interventions to help achieve those expected outcomes. You'll also set objective criteria to evaluate the effectiveness of your interventions.

Can I read that back to you?

Be sure to double-check, clarify or restate the information you've collected to make sure that it's accurate and complete. Validating the data helps you avoid misinterpretation. Remember, if your assessment is incorrect or incomplete, the nursing diagnoses you formulate are likely to be incorrect as well or you may overlook a problem and neglect to formulate a diagnosis for it.

Also, to make sure that the data you've gathered accurately reflects the patient's life experiences and living patterns, maintain an objective, non-judgemental approach during assessment.

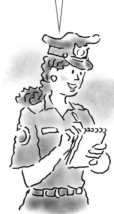

Think of the nursing assessment as a fact-finding mission.

Complete vs. focused assessment

Depending on the situation and time constraints, your assessment may be complete or focused.

You complete me

A *complete* assessment provides comprehensive baseline information. Typically, it's conducted when the patient is admitted. Student nurses are generally expected to perform a complete assessment as part of their learning experience.

Hocus focus

A *focused* assessment generally is problem- or need-orientated. During this assessment, focus on evaluating for specific problems or concerns that have already been identified and are being tracked by the health care team until they're resolved.

Typically, you'll perform a focused assessment when the patient is first admitted, at the beginning of a shift, whenever the patient has a new complaint or a change in condition or when you're evaluating the results of an intervention.

What did the care plan say to the assessment findings? You complete me!

Components of a complete health assessment

A complete and holistic health assessment includes the:
- health history
- physical, psychological, social and spiritual assessment
- consideration of laboratory and diagnostic test results
- review of other available health information.

First impressions

Assessment begins as soon as you meet your patient. Perhaps without even being aware of it, you're already noting such aspects as their skin colour, speech patterns and body position. Your education as a nurse gives you the ability to organise and interpret this data. As you move on to conduct the formal nursing assessment, you'll collect data in a more structured way. The findings you collect from your assessment may be subjective or objective. (See *Subjective vs. objective findings*, page 22.)

Group dynamics

When evaluating the assessment data, you'll start to recognise significant points and ask pertinent questions. You'll probably find yourself starting

Teacher knows best

Subjective vs. objective findings

Keep in mind that assessment findings fall into two broad categories: subjective and objective.

Subjective data

Subjective assessment data represents the perception or reality experienced by the person reporting the information. It may come directly from the patient or indirectly from family members, caregivers or other health care providers. For example, when you ask a patient to rate his pain on a scale of 0 to 10, you're asking him to quantify his personal perception of the severity of his pain. Even indirect data can provide clues that could prove vital to your patient's care. In some cases—for instance, if your patient is physically or mentally incapable of answering questions or providing information—such third-party sources are crucial to your assessment.

Objective data

Objective data come from the physical examination and assessment of the patient. Use physical findings to verify the subjective findings you've gathered from the patient's health history. For example, a temperature of 38.5°C (objective data) supports the patient's report of 'feeling hot and bothered' (subjective data).

to group related bits of significant assessment data into clusters that give you clues about your patient's problem and prompt additional questions. For instance, if the data suggest a pattern of poor nutrition, you should ask questions that will help elicit the cause, such as:
- Can you describe your appetite?
- Do you eat most meals alone?
- Do you have enough money to buy food?

On the other hand, if the patient reports frequent nausea, you should suspect that this may be the cause of his poor nutrition. Therefore, you'd ask questions to elicit more information about this symptom, such as:
- Do you feel nauseated after meals? Before meals?
- Do any of your medications upset your stomach?

History

The nursing history requires you to collect information about the patient's:
- biographical data
- current physical and emotional complaints
- past medical history

- past and current ability to perform activities of daily living (ADLs)
- availability of support systems, effectiveness of past coping patterns and perceived stressors
- socioeconomic factors affecting preventive health practices and concordance with medical recommendations
- spiritual and cultural practices, wishes or concerns
- family patterns of illness.

Biographical data

Begin your history by obtaining biographical data from the patient. Do this before you begin gathering details about his health. Ask the patient their name, address, telephone number, birth date, age, marital status, religion and nationality. Find out who the patient lives with and get the name and number of a person to contact in case of an emergency. Also ask the patient about their health care, including the name of their general practitioner and any other health care professionals or members of the interprofessional team they have contact with, for example an asthma nurse specialist or social worker.

If the patient can't give accurate information, ask for the name of a friend or relative who can. Always document the source of the information you collect as well as whether an interpreter was necessary and present.

Current complaints

To explore the patient's current complaints, ask the patient about the circumstances that have brought them into contact with the health care team. Is there an aspect of their health that is concerning them or proving challenging? Patient complaints provide valuable data immediately. When you explore these initial complaints, you may uncover crucial additional information.

Digging in the dirt

Record the patient's complaints in their own words. Ask them to describe the problem in detail, including any suspected cause. Keep in mind that, in many cases, presenting signs and symptoms are the tip of the iceberg. You must use your skills and knowledge to uncover facts about what's really going on. Obtaining a thorough patient history is one way to do this.

Past medical history

Ask the patient about past and current medical problems. Typical questions include:
- Have you ever been hospitalised? If so, when and why?
- Did you have any childhood illnesses?

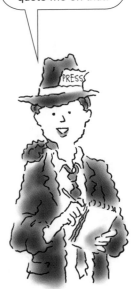

Recording your patient's complaints in their own words is good nursing practice. You can quote me on that!

- Are you currently being treated for any problem, such as hypertension or diabetes? If so, for what problem and who is treating you?
- Have you ever had surgery? If so, when and why?
- Are you allergic to anything in the environment or to any drugs or foods? If so, what kind of allergic reaction do you have? Do you have any sensitivities that you know of?
- Are you taking medications, including over-the-counter (OTC) preparations, such as aspirin, vitamins or cough syrup? If so, how much do you take and how often do you take it? Do you use home remedies such as homemade ointments? Do you use herbal preparations or take dietary supplements? Do you use other alternative or complementary therapies, such as acupuncture, massage, or reiki?
- Do you have any pain? If so, how would you rate your pain on a 0-to-10 pain scale? What aggravates or relieves your pain? How long have you had it?

Activities of daily living

Find out about your patient's ability to perform ADLs by asking them to describe his typical day. The types of information you seek should include:

- appetite, special diets, food allergies and meal preparation
- urinary and bowel elimination habits
- exercise and sleep habits and any aids required for sleep
- work and leisure activities
- use of tobacco, alcohol and other drugs.

Also be sure to elicit the patient's view of how the present illness has affected their usual performance of ADLs.

Support systems and stressors

Because illness doesn't occur in isolation, you also need to ask about other aspects of your patient's life, including the availability of support systems and perceived stressors, when you collect your history data. These other life factors can enhance or complicate a patient's condition or affect his recovery.

Thank you for being a friend

For instance, lack of social support can affect a patient's physical well-being and influence patient outcomes. In addition to family members, a patient's social support system may include friends, co-workers, community groups and church members who provide assistance in times of anxiety or crisis.

You can begin your evaluation of your patient's support system by asking the patient, 'Who's with you today?' or 'How did you get here today?' Other questions that elicit information about the patient's support system include:

- Is anyone available to help you at home, if needed?
- Who would you want to be involved in your care?
- Who are the people that are important to you?

More intimate details of the patient's social support system are usually best obtained in ongoing interactions during care giving activities or as you and the patient begin to discuss discharge plans. As appropriate, weave the information you obtain about your patient's support system into the care plan.

Stress marks

Emotional, social and physical demands on the body cause stress. The amount of stress a patient experiences can affect their physiological and psychological health. To elicit information about your patient's stress level and methods of coping with stress, ask:

- what situations they find stressful
- how they respond physically to stress
- what they do when they feel stress
- whether stress affects family relationships
- if they think stress affects their health.

Also, inquire about potential stressors, such as recent bereavements or changes in circumstances, spiritual concerns, difficulties with self-care or normal ADLs and exposure to abuse (see *Asking about abuse*). These may be important clues that help you formulate a care plan.

Asking about abuse

A history of abuse is an important aspect of a patient's psychosocial history. Remember that anyone can be a victim of abuse, including a boyfriend or girlfriend, a spouse, an elderly person, a child or a parent. In addition, abuse can occur in many forms, including physical, psychological, emotional and sexual abuse.

When taking a health history, you should ask two questions to explore abuse:

- When do you feel safe?
- When do you not feel safe?

Reaction time

Even when you don't immediately suspect an abusive situation, be aware of how your patient reacts to open-ended questions. Is the patient defensive, hostile, confused or frightened? Assess how the patient interacts with you and others. Does he or she seem withdrawn or frightened or show other inappropriate behaviour? Keep his or her reactions in mind when you perform your physical assessment.

Remember to report

Remember, if the patient tells you about any type of abuse, you may be obligated to report it and you should always inform the patient that this is what you are going to do. Be guided by the Nursing and Midwifery Council (NMC) Code of Conduct, and legislation related to the protection of children and vulnerable adults and local policies and procedures. If in doubt ask for advice from a senior member of staff!

Socioeconomic factors

The patient's socioeconomic status can directly affect health behaviours by determining the financial resources available for health care and a healthy lifestyle, including adequate housing, clothing and nutrition. For example, a patient whose financial resources barely meet basic needs is less likely to use services or products designed to promote or maintain health. To assess health-related socioeconomic factors, find out if your patient has a regular income and whether they are receiving any kind of benefits. Try to establish whether his or her income is sufficient to pay for housing, food and clothing.

Spiritual and cultural influences

Some patients attach great importance to their spiritual and religious beliefs. Spirituality (one's personal definition of the purpose and meaning of life and the world) may assign meaning to individual and community life, guide daily behaviour and lifestyle, define acceptable health care and influence attitudes toward illness and death.

Divine thing

Religion is the component of spirituality that includes particular practices related to a belief in a divine power. A religious system usually embraces more specific beliefs, including prescribed behaviours, rituals or practices. A patient's health beliefs and practices may be linked closely to religion, for example whether or not a blood transfusion is seen as acceptable.

Culture club

A patient's cultural background can also profoundly influence his views of life and death, health beliefs, health and dietary habits, roles, relationships and family dynamics. For example, patients from some cultures avoid seeking health care or taking responsibility for changing unhealthy behaviours because they feel powerless to control their illness, which they may consider punishment for some wrongdoing. To find out about your patient's spiritual and cultural influences, ask these questions:
• Do you have religious or cultural beliefs that affect your diet or health practices?
• Would you like me to contact any religious group for you?
   Assessing cultural influences can bring health-related factors to light and identify culturally related strengths, such as a strong support system.

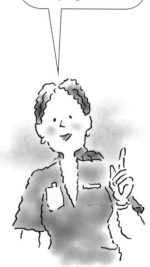

When assessing your patient's spiritual beliefs, don't let your own beliefs colour your attitude. Remember to remain nonjudgemental.

Lost in translation?

If the patient has a language barrier, talk with your manager or the family to assist you in finding an interpreter. When you first interact with the patient with an interpreter present, explain basic routines and establish a functional method of communicating about important health issues, such as pain, constipation, nausea or other common symptoms. This is also a good time to verify that the patient understands use of the call bell and any treatments or restrictions ordered. Family members can also be used as interpreters but be aware that this may affect the way in which information is translated.

Show a little respect

Being observant, open and interested is commonly the best way to learn about other people's spiritual and cultural viewpoints. Whether you're asking questions or responding to patient queries, be careful to avoid making assumptions about people who might be ethnically or culturally different from you. A simple opening question such as, 'Would you be comfortable if I …?' can demonstrate your respect for the patient's feelings and your willingness to adapt your care to the patient's needs.

Family history

Questioning the patient about his family's health is a good way to uncover his risk of having certain illnesses. (See *All in the family history*.)

All in the family history

Being aware of patterns of illness in families can help you understand genetic risk factors, determine the influence of these events on the attitudes of your patient and plan effective interventions. For example, a 49-year-old male with a family history of several male deaths from heart attack before age 50 who experiences chest pain may be significantly more afraid than a peer with a similar complaint but no early male cardiac deaths in his family.

In some clinical settings, you may not have access to a family medical history because it's obtained by the doctor but isn't immediately available to you. In this case, obtain a brief history of relevant illness in the patient's parents, siblings and, when indicated, grandparents. Typical questions include:

- Are your mother, father and siblings living?
- If not, how old were they when they died? What were the causes of their deaths?
- If they're alive, do they have diabetes, high blood pressure, heart disease, asthma, cancer, sickle cell anaemia, haemophilia, cataracts, glaucoma or other illnesses?

Physical examination

During the physical examination, you obtain data using your five senses—sight, hearing, touch, smell and feel. A complete examination includes a general survey, measurement of vital signs, height and weight measurements and assessment of all organs and body systems. (See *Examining the goals of a physical examination*.) Of course, in many cases, you won't have time for a complete examination and will need to focus on particular complaints or health problems.

General survey

The general survey provides vital information about the patient's behaviour and health status. During your first contact with the patient, expect to receive a steady stream of impressions—most of which are visual. The patient's sex, race and approximate age will usually be obvious. Because some health concerns may relate to these factors, be sure to note them.

Also note less-obvious factors that can contribute to an overall impression, including:
- signs of distress
- facial characteristics
- body type, posture and movements
- speech
- dress
- grooming and personal hygiene
- style of interacting with others.

Teacher knows best

Examining the goals of a physical examination

During the physical examination, keep in mind that your goal as a nurse is to identify signs, symptoms and problems for which the patient needs nursing interventions. In other words, the data you collect should lead you to formulate a nursing diagnosis—not a medical diagnosis. The nurse's focus is always on patient processes.

Doctors, on the other hand, use a method called *differential diagnosis* to arrive at a medical diagnosis. After identifying signs and symptoms, they systematically eliminate related diagnoses until they identify and substantiate a precise diagnosis by objective means, such as radiology or laboratory findings. The doctor's focus is on the disease processes.

Meaningful collaboration amongst doctors and nurses leads to health care that maximises the patient's health and quality of life or preserves his comfort and dignity in death.

Summarise

When you've completed the survey, document your initial impressions of the patient in a one-paragraph statement—a summary that gives an overall picture to guide your subsequent examination.

Physical examination techniques

To perform the physical examination, you'll use a number of techniques, but will use predominantly inspection, observation and assessment skills.

All eyes on inspection

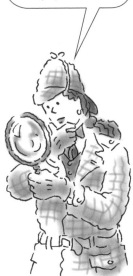

Don't forget that observation is an important part of the physical exam.

Inspection, or critical observation, is the most frequently used assessment technique. Performed correctly, it also reveals more than the other techniques. But incomplete or hasty inspection may neglect important details or yield false or misleading findings.

To ensure accurate, useful information, approach inspection in a careful, unhurried manner. It is often best to start with a basic set of observations (for example, blood pressure, pulse, respiratory rate and temperature) before moving on to other more focused assessments. Pay close attention to details as you assess each body system, using all of your senses and observing for colour, size, location, movement, texture, symmetry, odours and sounds. Try to draw logical conclusions from the findings. You should also make use of relevant assessment tools, for example a pressure ulcer risk assessment, a mobility assessment or a nutritional screening tool. Remember that you are also establishing baselines that can be used to measure whether a patient's condition is improving, worsening or remaining the same.

Diagnostic testing data

Make sure that you know how to access the patient's laboratory and other diagnostic test results. In most record-keeping systems, laboratory results are printed or electronically formatted on forms that specify what laboratory performed the test, the normal range of values for that test, the patient's test value and where that value lies in relation to the normal range.

Other test results may be filed by type or located by date of service. Radiology, nuclear scanning, computed tomography (CT), magnetic resonance imaging and ultrasound results are commonly kept together. Endoscopic and biopsy reports may be filed separately, with the report containing a section on the procedure process as well as the specific findings. Electrocardiograms are commonly kept together for ease of comparison.

Supporting role

Nurses not only need to be aware of what tests the patient has had and the results, but should have an understanding of the disease process and what these results may mean. Patients may be understandably anxious about the details of preparing for or going through a particular test, how soon the results will be available and what these results mean. The nurse is responsible for teaching and preparing the patient and then identifying and responding to post-test complications or reactions. The doctor is usually responsible for conveying test results and implications to the patient, but nurses are commonly asked to review and clarify the information provided as the patient thinks through what he has been told.

Other health information in the patient's notes

The patient's notes are an excellent source of assessment data. Always review documentation carefully, including assessments made by other health care team members, such as accident and emergency staff, the admitting doctor, consulting medical specialists, other nursing staff, dieticians, physiotherapists, pharmacists or social workers. The doctor's history and physical examination findings can guide your questioning during assessment. If appropriate, you should attempt to corroborate these findings during the nursing assessment. If your assessment findings differ, report your findings as appropriate.

Medication use

Be sure to review your patient's current medication use. Ask about prescription drugs, OTC drugs and herbal remedies. List these medications on the patient's chart when he's admitted. Medications that are prescribed during hospitalisation should be listed on a medication administration record (MAR). Look closely at the details of each drug order.

Look before you leap

Before your first patient contact, check your patient's list of prescribed drugs and their dosages and make sure that you know what adverse reactions and interactions these drugs could cause. Find out if the patient understands the purpose of each drug; this will help determine if he needs additional teaching during hospitalisation or at discharge. If appropriate, ask about the patient's previous medication use as well, find out if he experienced adverse reactions, and ask about recreational drug use.

If you question a drug, dosage or route listed on the MAR, double-check the prescription first, and then call the pharmacy, doctor or prescriber as appropriate. In the community, check the labels on the patient's prescriptions and call the pharmacy or the general practitioner to validate discrepancies between the labels, the patient's statements and the doctor's orders in the drug chart.

Overdose of drug data

For educational purposes, lecturers commonly ask students to explore medications typical to the patients they will find in each clinical placement, so for example the drugs used to treat diabetes, prior to a medical placement. (See *Everything you always wanted to know about drugs but were afraid of forgetting* and *Resources for reliable drug information*, pages 32 and 33.)

> Get to know your patient's medication list inside and out. It may affect your care plan. Getting to know you.

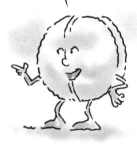

Everything you always wanted to know about drugs but were afraid of forgetting

To help you learn and retain important information about the multitude of drugs you'll be administering, you should consider developing your own database that covers the drugs you will typically see being used. Here are suggestions for the types of information you might collect on each drug and a sample entry.

Information required	Example
Generic name (trade name)	• Lisinopril (Carace, Zestril)
Class (pharmacological, therapeutic, or both)	• *Pharmacological:* angiotensin-converting enzyme (ACE) inhibitor • *Therapeutic:* antihypertensive
Action	• Lowers blood pressure by suppressing the renin–angiotensin–aldosterone system • Blocks the enzyme that converts angiotensin I to angiotensin II, which also decreases aldosterone production • Causes decreased blood pressure from less vasoconstriction, a small increase in potassium and some sodium and fluid loss
Dose (normal and patient's)	• *Normal:* initially, 10 mg daily when patient is also on a thiazide diuretic; usual effective dosage 20–40 mg daily; maximum dosage 80 mg daily
Specific therapeutic use (this patient)	• Lower blood pressure to below 120/80 mmHg because diuretic alone was insufficient
Contraindications and precautions	• Contraindicated in patients hypersensitive to or with a history of angioedema from ACE inhibitors • Contraindicated in women who are in their last two trimesters of pregnancy • Use cautiously in patients with impaired renal function (may need to adjust dose) • Use cautiously in patients at risk for hyperkalemia, heart failure (use only when other drugs are ineffective) or salt or volume depletion • Use cautiously in women who are breast-feeding • Rare but life-threatening adverse reactions: hyperkalemia, angioedema, anaphylaxis, pancytopenia
Major adverse effects	• Common adverse reactions: dizziness, fatigue, headache, insomnia: nasal congestion; diarrhoea, nausea; muscle cramps; dry, persistent, tickling, non-productive cough (most common reason for stopping drug due to side effects)
Drug or food interactions	• Diuretics: may cause excessively low blood pressure • Potassium-sparing diuretics, potassium supplements: may increase risk of hyperkalemia • Thiazide diuretics: may decrease potassium loss caused by these diuretics • Insulins, oral antidiabetics: may increase risk of hypoglycaemia
Effects on laboratory test results	• May increase potassium, blood urea nitrogen, serum creatinine and liver function test levels, including bilirubin

(continued)

Everything you always wanted to know about drugs but were afraid of forgetting (continued)

Information required	Example
Nursing implications	• Monitor for adverse effects and drug interactions • Give orally without regard to meals (although use with meals may decrease gastrointestinal [GI] adverse effects) • Determine if the patient is pregnant or may become pregnant. Notify the doctor as needed and tell the patient of the risks
Patient teaching	• Teach the patient to immediately call or see a doctor or nurse if swelling of eyes, face, lips or tongue with difficulty breathing appears (most common with first dose of drug) • Instruct the patient that light-headedness may occur, especially during the first few days of treatment; to rise slowly to avoid this effect; to notify the doctor and to stop the drug and call the doctor promptly if fainting occurs • Tell the patient to watch for signs of infection, such as fever, sore throat, productive cough and poorly healing wounds and to notify the doctor if any of these signs occur • Teach women of child-bearing age to use effective contraception and to stop the drug if pregnancy occurs • Inform the patient of the importance of regular blood pressure monitoring and laboratory testing by the practitioner. Also, teach about the use of a home blood pressure monitoring device, if appropriate

Resources for reliable drug information

The British National Formulary (BNF)

The BNF is the most commonly used source of information on drugs. It contains information on all medications that are licensed for use in the United Kingdom, including prescription-only and OTC medications. The BNF is updated every six months, and there is also a *BNF for children*. Copies of the BNF should be available in all clinical areas, and should be referred to regularly by those prescribing and administering medications. Student nurses will find the BNF a particularly useful resource for learning about the administration of medications.

Over-the-counter drugs, herbs and supplements

Information on all OTC drugs, herbs and supplements (including vitamins and minerals) might not appear in the BNF. However, you'll need good resource material about these products. The fact that they're readily available leads some of these products to be dangerously used and abused. Some patients assume that if a drug or herbal remedy is sold without a prescription, it's completely safe to use, even overuse, regardless of the warnings on the label. A good resource can help you determine all the risks of improper use, expand your understanding of potential adverse effects, alert you to potential interactions

(continued)

Resources for reliable drug information (continued)

with other drugs and herbs and help you plan patient teaching.

Nurses, pharmacists and prescribers need to keep up-to-date with the latest research on herbal preparations, including what medical conditions can be helped by various herbs, what dosages appear to be beneficial, what dosages appear to be toxic and what adverse effects or drug interactions might occur. Being attuned to good sources of reliable information can assist you in caring for your patients.

Finding reliable references

When researching drug information, remember to check the date of publication. Many nursing and practitioner references are updated yearly, but not all. Drug product labels are only updated when new indications or dosage forms are approved or new warnings are required.

The resources listed here are available to provide you with reliable drug and herb information.

Prescription drugs

- The drug product label is a valid source of approved information.
- Companies that manufacture older generic drugs may no longer make the drug product label readily available. Reputable online pharmacy web sites, such as *www.drugs.com* and *www.rxlist.com*, are good sources of information about these products.
- Several pharmacist- and practitioner-orientated drug reference books, such as *Facts and Comparisons*, can generally be found in your University library. These resources usually provide more-accessible formats and a wider range of information than product labels.
- Many nurses prefer to use a nursing drug reference book for day-to-day information geared to their needs. Such books as the *Nursing Drug Handbook* (and companion web site *www.NDHnow.com*) or *Springhouse Nurse's Drug Guide* (geared toward students) can be invaluable for checking nursing considerations and patient teaching information in addition to providing essential information on indications, dosages, contraindications and cautions, therapeutic and pharmacologic effects and adverse reactions.
- Specialty references, such as *Dangerous Drug Interactions* by Lippincott Williams & Wilkins and *Patient Drug Facts* by Facts & Comparisons, can also be useful in developing teaching plans.

Herbal products

- *The Review of Natural Products* by Facts & Comparisons, which may be available in your school library, is an example of a reliable publication from providers of prescription information.
- The nursing-based resource *Nursing Herbal Medicine Handbook* provides nursing considerations and patient-teaching information in addition to the standard information.

Medical procedure data

Review the medical procedures scheduled for your patient. Knowing which procedures the patient is scheduled for can help you anticipate potential problems and alert you to postprocedure signs and symptoms to watch for.

For example . . .

If the patient is scheduled for surgery, you would expect to verify the allergy history, looking particularly for an allergy to iodine or other contrast materials, and notify the doctor and anaesthetists of any new information. You would also expect to explain to the patient what's going to happen before, during and after the procedure, including transfer to theatres, and educate them about procedure restrictions, including the need to:

- withhold solid foods and certain medications before the surgery
- shower and put on theatre gown
- remove any jewellery or prostheses
- empty bladder and possibly bowels before surgery.

Similarly, if the patient has just undergone a procedure involving other medications, you would know to assess for adverse reactions to these agents.

Admitting medical diagnosis

You should also review the patient's medical diagnosis. Determine if your patient's current complaints and assessment findings match his admitting diagnosis. If you uncover new information, report it to the doctor because these new findings may affect the treatment plan. Make sure you understand the meaning and implications of your patient's medical diagnosis—including its pathophysiology, signs and symptoms, required diagnostic tests, treatments, complications, preparation for procedures and postprocedure care. This information helps you focus your assessment.

Special consideration

If your patient is diagnosed with ulcerative colitis, for instance, you would realise that he's more prone to develop anaemia due to internal bleeding. Consequently, you would be sure to monitor his haematology reports, check his vital signs frequently and observe elimination patterns and changes. On the other hand, for a patient admitted with type-one diabetes, you would stay alert for signs and symptoms of hypoglycaemia or hyperglycaemia.

Data collection and organisation

Every nurse must know how to collect and organise patient data in a meaningful format. Doing this helps you formulate correct nursing diagnoses and allows other health care team members to readily understand the data you've documented.

As part of your nurse education and as a way of developing your care planning skills, you may be asked to organise your information by using a particular framework. In the clinical setting, many different types of integrated or speciality assessment formats may be used, according to the regulations and specific requirements for that area. These frameworks for organising and managing assessment information are often linked to nursing models based on the work of people such as Roper, Logan and Tierney (their 12 ADLs are very popular!), Orem, Roy or Peplau. As well as providing a framework for organising the delivery of care, these nursing models can specify the underlying philosophy for the way in which the care should be delivered.

Data should be collected and organised in a methodical and structured way, and it should be guided by the documentation in use in each clinical area. However, the most important thing to remember is that regardless of whichever nursing model or assessment framework is being utilised, care planning always involves following the stages of the nursing process. If you stick with the nursing process you can apply your skills to whichever environment you are working in, and you can't go wrong!

Gordon's functional health patterns

To organise and analyse the patient data you collect, you may want to use the functional health patterns and rating scale proposed in 1987 by Marjory Gordon. Gordon's functional health categories include:
- health perception and management
- nutrition and metabolism
- elimination
- activity and exercise
- cognition and perception
- sleep and rest
- self-perception and self-concept
- sexuality and reproduction
- roles and relationships
- coping and stress management
- values and beliefs.

These 11 categories provide a framework for a systematic, standardised approach to data collection.

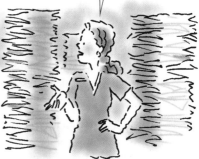

The data you collect on your patient can be overwhelming. Good thing that there are systems for organising all these data.

You can use Gordon's functional health patterns to obtain a nursing history from the patient's perspective through a series of specific questions. These patterns are flexible and adaptable and can be used for patients in various states of health, from different age-groups and in different clinical settings. By focussing on each health pattern in turn, you can better evaluate your patient's overall level of health and well-being. You can also establish what is normal for your patient and how their health status has changed.

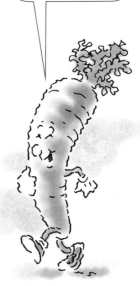

Gordon says that nutrition and metabolism are one of the 11 functional health categories.

Health perception and management

To obtain data about the health perception and management pattern, ask questions that help determine the patient's:
- perception of his level of health
- detrimental habits, such as smoking or excessive alcohol use
- actual or potential problems related to safety and health management or the need for home modifications or continuing care at home.

Activity and exercise

When evaluating the patient's activity and exercise pattern, assess:
- the patient's ability to manage normal ADLs that require energy expenditure, including self-care, exercise and leisure time
- major body systems involved with activity and exercise (respiratory, cardiovascular and musculoskeletal systems).

Nutrition and metabolism

To assess nutrition and metabolism, ask the patient questions about:
- food and fluid consumption relative to metabolic needs
- adequacy of nourishment
- dietary habits and preferences, and influencing factors, including financial constraints and access to shops
- problems related to fluid balance, tissue integrity and adequate nutrition
- GI problems.

Elimination

To assess your patient's elimination pattern, ask questions related to his excretory patterns (bowel, bladder and skin) and check for such problems as incontinence, constipation, diarrhoea and urinary retention.

Sleep and rest

When assessing the patient's sleep and rest pattern, inquire about:
- normal sleep, rest and relaxation practices
- dysfunctional sleep patterns, fatigue and responses to sleep deprivation.

Cognition and perception

To assess cognition and perception, evaluate the patient's:
- ability to comprehend and use information
- sensory and neurological functions
- sensory experiences, such as pain and altered sensory input.

Self-perception and self-concept

To assess your patient's self-perception and self-concept, evaluate:
- attitudes toward self, including identity, body image, self-worth, and self-esteem
- response to threats to self-concept.

Sexuality and reproduction

To assess the patient's sexuality and reproduction pattern, evaluate:
- satisfaction or dissatisfaction with sexuality patterns and reproductive functions
- sexuality concerns.

Roles and relationships

To assess your patient's roles and relationships, evaluate:
- roles in the world and relationships with others
- satisfaction with roles
- role strain
- dysfunctional relationships.

Coping and stress management

Explore your patient's coping and stress management pattern by asking questions about his:
- perception of stress and coping strategies
- support systems

- symptoms of stress
- effectiveness of coping strategies in terms of stress tolerance.

Values and beliefs

To assess the patient's values and beliefs, evaluate:
- religious or spiritual orientation
- goals and values that guide decisions.

Integrated and specialty database formats

For consistency, most clinical areas require that staff document assessment findings using standardised formats. Typically, history and physical findings are on the same form and it may form part of an integrated care pathway. The purpose of using a standardised format is to provide a comprehensive, consistent, understandable framework for nursing data. Standardised formats enhance information exchange and communication among staff members and, when necessary, among health care providers. However, when a standardised format is used, nurses typically adapt their assessment techniques to the flow of the form. (See *Integrated admission database form*, pages 38 to 41.)

Custom or generic?

Some clinical areas use assessment forms customised for their particular needs; others use more generic forms. Often the same forms will be used throughout an acute or primary care trust. Some standardised forms are designed to promote closer monitoring and evaluation of patient status trends, patterns and longitudinal observations and changes. They're especially useful in critical care areas, where the patient's status can change in mere moments.

Digital age

Health care providers are increasingly using computerised care plans. As a nursing student, you're probably familiar with the use of these in some clinical settings, but expect to need time to adapt to integrating usage of these into your patient care.

Speciality assessments

Your patient's age and health status may require you to perform a more specialised examination, using an appropriately focused assessment tool. Specialised assessment tools include the Glasgow Coma Scale, pain rating scales, Mini-Mental Status Examination, and pressure ulcer risk assessments. The most common specialised assessments are those used for specific populations, such as paediatric, elderly, maternal and psychiatric patients, or particular areas of concern, for example skin integrity, nutrition or pain.

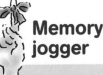

Memory jogger

To remember Gordon's functional patterns, think of the slogan 'Hey Nurse! Every Action Can Start, Stimulate, Stop or Reverse your Care Victory!'

Health perception and management
Nutrition and metabolism
Elimination
Activity and exercise
Cognition and perception
Sleep and rest
Self-perception and self-concept
Sexuality and reproduction
Roles and relationships
Coping and stress management
Values and beliefs.

Integrated admission database form

Most health care facilities use a multidisciplinary admission form. The sample form below has spaces that can be filled in by the nurse, doctor and other members of the interprofessional team.

Name _Beatrice Perry_

Address _2 Clayton Street_

Bourne, Lincs 01555 020972

Admission Date _2_ / _26_ / _01_ Time _1345_

Admitted per: ____ Ambulatory

_✔_ Stretcher ____ Wheelchair

T _97_ P _92_ R _24_ BP _98_ / _52_

Ht. _5'2"_ Wt. _225 lb_

(estimated/(actual))

SECTION COMPLETED BY: _P. Lippman, CST_ **TIME:** _1350_

ORIENTATION TO ROOM/UNIT
POLICIES EXPLAINED

✔ Call light
✔ Bed oper.
✔ Phone
✔ Television
✔ Meals
___ Advance directive explained
___ Living will

___ Living will on chart
___ Valuables form completed
✔ Elec.
✔ Smoking
___ Side rails
✔ ID bracelet on
___ Visiting hours

Name and phone numbers of two people to call if necessary:

NAME	RELATIONSHIP	PHONE #
Mary Ryan	_daughter_	_0111-120119_
Thomas Perry	_son_	_02222-424424_

REASON FOR HOSPITALISATION ____ (patient quote:) _I go numb in my (R) arm and leg_

ANTICIPATED DATE OF DISCHARGE: _28/02/09_

PREVIOUS HOSPITALISATIONS: SURGERY/ILLNESS

THA   DATE _15/01/01_

HEALTH PROBLEM	Yes	No	?
Arthritis		✔	
Blood problem (anemia, sickle cell, clotting, bleeding)		✔	
Cancer		✔	
Diabetes	✔		
Eye problems (cataracts, glaucoma)		✔	
Heart problem		✔	
Liver problem		✔	
Hiatal hernia		✔	
High blood pressure	✔		
HIV/AIDS		✔	
Kidney problem		✔	
Comments:			

HEALTH PROBLEM	Yes	No	?
Lung problem ((Emphysema) Asthma, Bronchitis, TB, Pneumonia, Shortness of breath)	✔		
Stroke		✔	
Ulcers		✔	
Thyroid problem		✔	
Psychological disorder		✔	
Alcohol abuse		✔	
Drug abuse			
Drug(s)			
		✔	
Smoking	✔		
Other			

ALLERGIES: ☐ TAPE ☐ IODINE ☐ LATEX ☐ no known allergies

☐ FOOD: _____ ✔ DRUG: _Penicillin - Rash_

☐ BLOOD REACTION: _____ ☐ OTHER: _____

MEDICATIONS: _____

HERBAL
PREPARATIONS: _____

INFORMATION RECEIVED FROM: **SECTION COMPLETED BY:**

✔ Patient ☐ Relative _____ ☐ Friend _____ ☐ Other _____ _Jill O'Brien, RN_ Date _26/02/01_ Time _1405_

Integrated admission database form (continued)

All assessment sections are to be completed by a professional nurse.   Date _28/02/01_

Patient name: _Beatrice Perry_
Record number: _554697_

GENERAL PHYSICAL APPEARANCE

✔ Clean _____ Disheveled

SKIN INTEGRITY: Indicate the location of any of the following on the chart to the right using the designated letter: a = rashes, b = lesions, c = significant bruises/abrasions, d = burns, e = pressure sores, f = recent scars, g = presence of tubes/appliances, h = other

Comments: _b ischemic leg ulcer (2 cm - healing)_

PRESSURE SORE POTENTIAL ASSESSMENT

PARAMETERS	0	1	2	3	Score
Mental status	(Alert)	Lethargic	Semicomatose (Count as double)	Comatose (Count as double)	0
Activity	Ambulatory	(Needs help)	Chairfast	Bedfast	1
Mobility	Full	(Limited)	Very limited	Immobile	1
Incontinence	(None)	Occasional	Usually of urine	Total of urine and feces	0
Oral nutrition intake	Good	(Fair)	Poor	None	1
Oral fluid intake	(Good)	Fair	Poor	None	0
Predisposing diseases (diabetes, neuropathies, vascular disease, anemias)	Absent	Slight	Moderate	(Severe)	3
Patients with scores of 10 or above should be considered at risk.				Total	6

FALL-RISK ASSESSMENT

Impaired: ____sensory function ____urinary/GI function ____mobility function ____mental status

____general debility/weakness
✔history of recent falls/dizziness/blackouts (automatically designates patient as prone-to-fall)
✔prone-to-fall risk (____✔____)

NEUROLOGICAL

____Dizziness ____Syncope ____Recent seizure ✔Numbness/tingling location: (R) arm and leg ____Headache ____Blurred vision

LOC: ✔Alert ____Lethargic ____Semicomatose ____Comatose
Mental Status: ✔Oriented ____Confused ____Disoriented
Speech: ✔Clear ____Slurred ____Garbled ____Aphasic

Neurological Checklist

	Right Arm	Left Arm	Right Leg	Left Leg	Right Pupil	Left Pupil	Pupil Reaction	Eyes Open	Best Verbal Response	Best Motor Response	Total
Coma Scale	+2/+4	+2/+4	5/6	↑	4	5	6	15			

Response	1	2	3	4	5	6
EYES OPEN	Never	To Pain	To Sound	Sponta-neously		
VERBAL	None	Incompre-hensible Sounds	Inappro-priate Words	Confused Conversa-tion	Oriented	
MOTOR	None	Extension	Flexion Abnormal	Flexion Withdrawal	Localizes Pain	

COMA SCALE CODE

+1:cannot move
+2:cannot move against gravity
+3:move against gravity
+4:move strongly against gravity

Comments: _numbness transient_   _T. Jones, MD_

CODE
Pupils: mm
Extremities movement/strength
Pupil Reaction
- Reactive
- Nonreactive
D Dilated
C Constricted
> Greater than
< Less than
= Equal
= Sluggish

1 2 3 4 5 6 7

BEHAVIORAL

Behavior: ✔Cooperative ____Uncooperative ____Depressed ____Restless ____Other ____Combative ✔Anxious ____Unresponsive

Comments: _____
Religious/Spiritual beliefs: _Lutheran_
Pt. request to contact minister/priest/rabbi? ✔Y ____N
Name _Rev. William Lacy_   Phone # _018-286-28403_

PAIN

Pt. having pain at present? ____Y ✔N
Pt. had pain in last several months? ____Y ✔N
Rate pain on a scale of 0-10 (0 = no pain, 10 = severe pain) _____
Pain location_____ Quality_____

Radiation____Y ____N Duration_____
What aggravates pain?_____What alleviates pain?_____
Effects on ADLs_____
Pt. pain goals _____

(continued)

Integrated admission database form (continued)

Patient name: _Beatrice Perry_
Record number: _554697_   Date _28/02/01_

CARDIOVASCULAR

Skin Color: ___Normal ___Flushed ___Pale ✔Cyanotic
Apical Pulse: ___Regular ✔Irregular ___Pacemaker: Type _____ Rate _____
Peripheral Pulses: ✔ Present ___Equal ✔ Weak ___Absent Comments: _bilat. weak lower extremities_
Specify: R___radial ___pedal L ___radial ___pedal
Comments: _____
Edema: ___No ✔Yes _+1 bilat. pretibial_ Numbness: ___No ✔Yes Site: _R arm and leg_
Chest Pain: ✔No ___Yes   P_____ Q_____ R_____ S_____ T_____
Family Cardiac History: ___No ✔Yes Telemetry Monitor: ___No ✔Yes rhythm _normal sinus_
Comments: _____

PULMONARY

Respirations: ✔Regular ___Irregular ___Shortness of breath ___Dyspnea on exertion
O₂ use at home? ___Yes ✔No
Chest expansion: ✔ Symmetrical ___Asymmetrical (explain: _____)
Breath sounds: ___Clear ___Crackles ___Rhonchi ✔ Wheezing Location _bilat upper lobe, inspiratory_
Cough: None ✔ Nonproductive ___Productive ___Describe _____
Comments: _pulse oximetry 98% on 2 L; sleeps with 2 pillows_

GASTROINTESTINAL

Stool:				
✔ Formed	Diarrhea ___		Obese ✔	*NUTRITION:
___ Loose	Constipation ___		thin ___	✔ Special Diet
___ Liquid	Abdomen:	✔ Soft	emaciated ___	_1800 ADA_
___ Mucus		✔ Rigid	nourished ___	___ Tube feeding
___ Ostomy		✔ Nontender		___ Chewing problem
___ Incontinent		___ Tender		___ Swallowing problems
Color: ✔ Brown		___ (Location)		___ Nausea/vomiting
___ Black	Bowel Sounds	✔ Present		___ Poor appetite
___ Red tinged		___ Absent		___ Wt. loss/gain ___ lb
___ Bloody		___ Hypoactive		
		___ Hyperactive		* Refer to dietitian if any ✔

GENITOURINARY/ REPRODUCTIVE

Color of Urine: ✔Yellow ___Amber ___Pink/Red tinged ___Brown ___Orange ___Clear ___Cloudy
___Ileo-Conduit ___Incontinent ___Catheter in place ___Frequency ___Urgency
___Difficulty in initiating stream ___Pain ___Burning ___Oliguria ___Anuria
___Dialysis   Access site: _____ Date of last dialysis: _____
Comments: _____
Date of LMP _1980_   Date of last PAP _5/00_   Breast self-exam ___Yes ✔No
Use of contraceptives: ___Yes (type _____) ___No ✔N/A
    Vaginal Discharge: ___Yes (describe _____) ✔No
    Bleeding: ___Yes (amount _____) ✔No
Pregnancies: Pregnant ___Yes ___Weeks gravida ___ Para ___ ✔No
Date of last Prostate Exam _____ Testicular self-exam ___Yes ___No
Comments: _____

ACTIVITY/ MOBILITY PATTERNS

___Ambulates independently ___Full ROM ___Limited ROM (explain: _____)
✔Ambulates with assistance (explain: _____) ✔cane ___walker ___crutches
___Gait steady/unsteady ___Mobility in bed (ability to turn self) _____
Musculoskeletal ___Pain___Weakness___Contractures___Joint swelling
___Paralysis___Deformity___Joint stiffness___Cast___Amputation
Describe: _____
Comments: _____

REST/ SLEEP PATTERNS

___Use of sleeping aids _____ Sleeps _6_ hr/day
Comments: _____

Additional assessment comment: _On arrival, diaphoretic and + hand tremors, vital signs stable, glucose 56 mg/dl._
Orange juice and lunch given to pt. 2 hr postprandial glucose 204 mg/dl. Symptoms subsided with juice. Nutritionist and di-
abetes educator consulted.   _Jill O'Brien, R.N._
MRI shows no cerebral lesions. Carotid Doppler ultrasound pending.   _B. Mayer, MD_

Integrated admission database form (continued)

EDUCATION/DISCHARGE SECTION
Instructions: Assessment sections must be completed within 8 hours of admission. Discharge planning and summary must be completed by day of discharge.

Patient name: _Beatrice Perry_
Record number: _554697_

EDUCATIONAL ASSESSMENT

Yes	No	
✔		Patient understands current diagnosis
✔		Family/significant other understands diagnosis
✔		Patient able to read English
✔		Patient able to write English
✔		Patient able to communicate
✔		Patient/family understands prehospital medication/treatment regimen

Yes	No	Emotional Factors:
✔		Patient appears to be coping*
✔		Family appears to be coping*
	✔	Any suspicion of family violence
	✔	Any suspicion of family abuse
	✔	Any suspicion of family neglect

Comment: _Diabetes teaching_

Language spoken, written, and read (other than English): _____
Interpreter services needed: ✔No ___Yes
Are there any barriers to learning (e.g., emotional, physical, cognitive)? _No_
Religious or cultural practices that may alter care or teaching needs? ___Yes ✔No Describe: _____
Is pt/family motivated to learn? ✔Yes ___No describe: _____

DISCHARGE ASSESSMENT

Living arrangements/caregiver (relationship): _Lives alone_
Type of dwelling: ___Apartment ✔House ___Nursing Home ___More than 1 floor? ✔Yes ___No Describe: _____
___Boarding Home ___Other _____
Physical barriers in home: ✔No ___Yes (explain): _____
Access to follow-up medical care: ✔Yes ___No (explain): _____
Ability to carry out ADLs: ___Self-care ✔Partial assistance ___Total assistance
Needs help with: ✔Bathing ___Feeding ___Ambulation ___Other
Anticipated discharge destination: ✔Home ___Rehab. ___Nursing Home ___SNF ___Boarding Home
___Other _____
Currently receiving services from a community agency? ___Yes ___No
If yes, check which one ___visiting nurses ___Meals on Wheels
Concerned about returning home? ___Being alone ___Financial problems ___Homemaking ___Meal prep.
___Managing ADLs ___Other _____

		Date		Time	
Assessment completed by:	_Jill O'Brien, R.N._	_28/02/01_		_1430_	
Assessment completed by:	_B. Mayer, MD_	_28/02/01_		_1445_	

DISCHARGE PLANNING

Resources notified:	Name	Date	Time	Signature
Social worker				
Home care coordinator	_M. Murphy, RN_	_28/02/01_	_0900_	_M. Murphy, RN_
Other				

Equipment/Supplies needed: _Stair chair_
Arranged for by: _M. Murphy, RN_ Date _28/02/01_ Time _0930_
Comment: _Daughter to stay with pt at home_

DISCHARGE SUMMARY

Alterations in patterns: If yes, explain.	Yes	No	Explanation
Nutrition	✔		_Adherence to ADA diet regimen_
Elimination		✔	
Self-care		✔	
Skin integrity		✔	
Mobility	✔		_Needs help with stairs_
Comfort pain		✔	
Mental status/behavior		✔	
Vision/Hearing/Speech		✔	

Discharge instructions given (specify): _Standard hosp. discharge instruction sheet_
Effects of illness on employment/lifestyle: _____
Central venous line removed: _N/A_ By whom: _____
Belongings sent with patient: ✔clothes ✔dentures ✔eyeglasses ___hearing aid ___prosthesis ___valuables
✔prescriptions ✔other _Cane_
Follow-up medical supervision to be provided by: _Dr. Schneider_
✔Patient/family instructed to call for follow-up appointment Discharge destination: _Pt's home with daughter_
Section completed by: _C. Rafferty, RN_ Date _28/02/01_ Time _1130_

You—the indispensable tool

Although standardised formats, specialised forms and computerised data collection enhance and promote information collection and health care delivery, you—the nurse—are the primary collector of patient data. No matter what format the clinical areas uses, data gathering and interpretation remain largely nursing responsibilities.

As a nurse, you're the ultimate—and indispensable—assessment tool. Not even the most sophisticated data collection tool or device can replace assessment by a skilled nurse.

Identifying growth and development stage

As children grow, they develop intellectually, morally, emotionally, sexually, socially and spiritually. They learn to think abstractly and logically, use language and explore the world around them. However, some theorists posit that growth and development don't end with childhood.

Erik H. Erikson is one of several theorists who explained how growth and development occur across the life span. As a part of your assessment documentation, your lecturers or mentors may ask you to identify which developmental stage your patient's growth represents. Although Erikson specifies an age range for each stage, don't be afraid to question whether your patient actually resembles a person facing the issues described. Some individuals may be mature beyond their years, while others may never have resolved the main crisis of a previous stage. Remember that you must be able to state why you believe your patient is moving through a particular stage. However, you aren't expected to be an expert in this area because you're still building your observation, listening and communication techniques. Becoming familiar with Erikson's theory, though, will help you identify and better understand your patient's psychosocial needs and may be helpful in planning a teaching strategy.

Eight is enough

According to Erikson, psychosocial development occurs in eight distinct stages, which he called 'the eight stages of man'. During each stage, a specific conflict occurs that the person must resolve. To resolve the conflict, the person undergoes a personality change, which gives him the strength to deal with the next developmental stage. If he can't resolve a conflict at a particular stage, he'll confront it later in life.

Stage 1: Trust vs. mistrust

During the first stage, which occurs from birth to about age 1, children develop trust if their needs are met. If their needs aren't met—or are met unpredictably—they become mistrustful.

Stage 2: Autonomy vs. shame and doubt

The second stage occurs between ages 1 and 3, when children learn to control their body functions and become increasingly independent. During this stage, they prefer to do things themselves and learn autonomy largely by imitating others. If they aren't allowed to be independent or are belittled for their efforts, they develop a sense of shame and self-doubt.

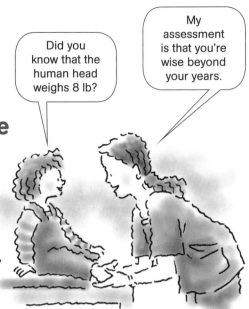

Stage 3: Initiative vs. guilt

During stage 3, which occurs between ages 3 and 6, children learn about the world through play and learn to cooperate with others. They develop a conscience and learn to balance their sense of initiative against the guilt they experience for doing something against their parents' wishes. If they fail this developmental stage, as adults they may be immobilised by guilt and continue to depend unduly on others.

Stage 4: Industry vs. inferiority

During stage 4, which occurs between ages 6 and 12, children enjoy working on projects and working with others. They tend to follow rules and become competitive. Social relationships take on great importance. If unrealistic expectations (or what they perceive as unrealistic expectations) are placed on them, they may develop feelings of inferiority. However, if they develop a sense of industry, they'll feel competent to meet life's expectations.

Stage 5: Identity vs. role confusion

From ages 12 to 18, adolescents experience rapid changes in their bodies. During this stage, they're preoccupied with how they look and how others view them. While trying to meet their peers' expectations, they also try to establish their own identity. If they fail to accomplish these tasks, they can suffer role confusion. If they navigate this stage successfully, they become confident adults who feel comfortable with who they are.

Stage 6: Intimacy vs. isolation

During this stage, young adults (ages 18 through 40) seek mutually satisfying relationships, including friends and marital partners. Many of them start families. Those who negotiate this stage successfully can experience intimacy on a deep level. Those who fail to do so become isolated and distant from others. Eventually, they may withdraw socially.

Stage 7: Generativity vs. self-absorption

During middle adulthood (ages 35 to 65), work and family take on great importance. People tend to be occupied with meaningful and creative work. They strive to contribute to the betterment of society and community, to transmit cultural values through the family and to establish a stable environment. As their children leave the home or their relationships or goals change, major life changes may occur and they struggle to find new meanings and purposes (commonly referred to as a *midlife crisis*). Failure to negotiate this stage successfully can lead to self-absorption and stagnation.

Stage 8: Integrity vs. despair

During late adulthood (ages 65 to death), people look back on their lives and accomplishments. If they have found a meaningful role in life, have a positive self-concept and can be intimate without strain, guilt or regret, they have a feeling of integrity. On the other hand, those who despair at their experiences and perceived failure may fear death as they struggle to find purpose in their lives.

Integrating assessment into care-giving tasks

The key to accomplishing multiple responsibilities in a short time is to view all patient care tasks as opportunities to uncover critical information. Every contact you have with a patient gives you an opportunity for assessment. Crucial information may come to light even during seemingly insignificant interactions. Answering the call bell, assisting with bathing, helping with range-of-motion exercises, even making casual conversation during bed-making and medication administration—these are all chances to observe the patient and gather valuable information.

Example

Suppose, for example, that you're beginning your shift. One of your patients is a 45-year-old woman who was admitted for cholecystectomy. The nurse presenting the handover report notes that the patient has been demanding and has been continually pressing the call bell. The patient's chart indicates that her vital signs have been stable, she has reported good pain control and she shows no signs of postoperative complications.

Dig deeper

Instead of simply accepting the 'demanding' label used by the exasperated nurse on the previous shift, you decide to investigate the patient's condition and seek more information, suspecting that the patient's behaviour could signal something deeper. Instead of waiting for the patient to press the call bell, you take the initiative to check on her frequently. Over the next 2 hours, the patient appears to become more relaxed.

> Remember that routine care giving tasks provide an opportune time to collect valuable assessment data.

You decide to use the opportunity of a morning bed bath to spend a little extra time with the patient and assess her emotional and psychological status. As the patient washes her face and upper body, you stand quietly by her side. After a few moments, you ask her how she feels about her recent surgery and her recovery so far. She confides that she's been upset with her care in the hospital and also doesn't know how she'll manage at home. She begins to talk about all the problems she's had since the gallbladder attack just before admission. You listen carefully as the patient finishes washing, interjecting occasionally to show her that you're paying attention. As you begin massaging her back with lotion at the end of the bed bath, the patient tearfully reveals that her husband passed away several weeks ago—important information about the patient that you didn't previously know. During the seemingly routine chore of meeting the patient's hygiene needs, you have obtained information that could prove crucial to the patient's recovery and follow-up care—information that could help you to create a more appropriate care plan for this frightened, grief-stricken patient.

Data uncovered

As you can see from the previous example, taking time to assess the patient as you perform other care giving tasks can help you to build rapport and uncover important patient information that may be crucial to your care plan.

Starting a concept map based on assessment data

In the university you attend, you gain a tremendous amount of knowledge. But do you wonder how to put this theoretical knowledge into practice, especially when you have to care for more than one or two patients? Do you wonder how to start a care plan from your assessment data? Let's look at a possible scenario.

Example

You're in your third year of training to be a children's nurse and are in your final placement at a small district hospital. At the start of the shift you're assigned to care for three patients on the children's ward, but before you even have chance to get started you learn you'll be receiving a new patient from accident and emergency. You look at your mentor, hoping that she'll step in to change your allocation of patients and find someone else to care for the new admission. Instead, she explains that this will be a good opportunity for you to expand your clinical skills and so two of your other three patients are reassigned to other nurses.

The paediatric patient from the accident and emergency, John Scott, arrives within minutes. You observe that he's anxious, crying and clinging to his mother, Christine Scott. The nurse handing over gives the following report:

The patient is an 8-year-old male who has had a high fever and severe stomach pain for the last 8 hours; abdominal guarding is present. Vital signs include temperature, 38.2 °C, heart rate 124 beats/minute, respiratory rate 28 breaths/minute, and blood pressure 132/80 mmHg. Complete blood count and blood chemistry samples have been sent to the laboratory, along with a urine specimen for urinalysis. The patient is scheduled for an emergency exploratory laparoscopy within the hour to rule out a ruptured appendix.

You note that the boy's mother seems shaken and holds her child closely. Before leaving, the accident and emergency nurse takes you aside and tells you the mother is worried about having to take time off from work because of this unexpected surgery. She hands you the patient's chart and leaves.

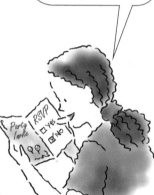

When asked to a panic party, turn down the invitation!

Don't push the panic button!

You're already running behind with your other patient. How can you possibly fulfil your nursing responsibilities to her and to your new patient? You need to admit the paediatric patient, introduce him to the hospital environment, assemble his chart, carry out the doctor's admitting orders, verify that the necessary consents have been signed, make sure that the laboratory test results are back and prepare the child (and his mother) for surgery. What's more, you need to perform an initial nursing assessment and then organise and document your findings before the boy goes to surgery so you can begin to develop a care plan. That's a tall order for a nursing student—or for *any* nurse. How would you handle it?

Chances are, you would feel overwhelmed, and your mind would race with frantic thoughts, such as: 'Yikes! I have way too much to do and not nearly enough time to do it! So much is expected of me—and so fast. How can I meet all these demands and still make sure that my other patient is safe and receives good care?'

Serenity now

Remember not to panic. You're only human and can't possibly do everything at once. Before you can attend to your duties, you must attend to yourself, so take time to calm down and collect yourself. One way to do this is to stop, look and listen. As a child, you were probably taught to stop, look and listen before crossing a street. The same procedure can help you focus when you find yourself in a stressful patient care situation. In this case, you stop first and then analyse what you've already looked at and listened to.

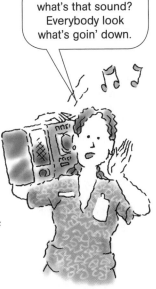

Stop, hey, what's that sound? Everybody look what's goin' down.

Stop sign

STOP stands for:
• **S**low down—Anxiety causes the release of adrenaline, a natural stimulant. (More stimulation is the last thing you need now!)
• **T**ake some deep breaths—However many it takes to calm down.
• **O**bjectify your feelings—That is, treat them impersonally; you don't have to deny them, but you can choose to not let them control your actions.
• **P**repare a plan and proceed professionally.
After you accomplish the first three steps, the last one will be much easier. A plan gives you structure and direction and can be especially reassuring when you're feeling stressed out.

You know more than you know

Once you 'stop' as described above, you'll find you feel less anxious, more in charge and better able to think like a professional. Now, you're ready to analyse and organise the information you've already looked at and listened to—namely, the impressions you started to form from the time you met the patient and his mother and heard the accident and emergency nurse's report. That's right—you've been gathering assessment information without really being aware of it.

Let's look at what you know so far:
• The patient is 8 years old.
• He has a high fever and is in pain.
• He has just been introduced to the strange sights, sounds, smells and people in the hospital and has just heard people talking about him rather than to him.
• He's old enough to understand what surgery is.
• He's emotionally upset, and his mother is upset as well.

As you begin your structured nursing assessment, you'll build on the developmental, emotional, physical and social information you've already collected.

Taking time for a concept map—what a concept!

Even in a hectic situation such as this, you might quickly sketch a concept map for yourself to help you focus on what you know and what you need to know. Utilising just the data you've been given and what you've observed, you can rough out a concept map. (See *Getting started*, page 48.)

Under construction

Getting started

Begin your concept map for the patient described in text by placing a circle in the centre of the page. In that circle, include the patient's name, age and medical diagnosis. Also note that his mother is present, and include her name.

When you have little information but you need a plan quickly, don't try to formulate nursing diagnoses for your concept map right off the bat. Instead, jot down main categories of problems as you think of them. For example, you might start by labelling a box 'GI symptoms' because you don't have enough information to get a handle on which nursing diagnoses are most appropriate. Include in this box any assessment findings that you collected from your observations and the shift report. Feel free to use abbreviations in your concept map (as shown below) to save time. Also, leave the boxes open so that you can add more information as you assess the patient and get his test results. You might not even want to draw connecting lines right away, but try to visualise the inter-relationships in your mind.

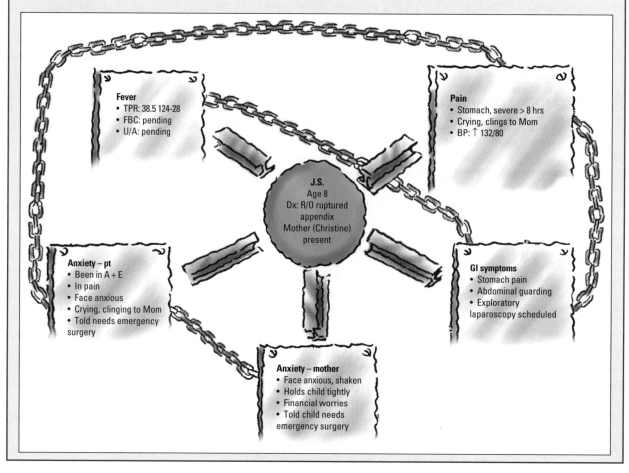

After you've gathered the patient assessment data, you're ready to move to the next step of the nursing process—formulating nursing diagnoses. As you learned in Chapter 1, creating a concept map helps you organise your thinking and see the big clinical picture.

On the case

Case study background

Benny Hayes, a 38-year-old male, was brought to the accident and emergency department after being involved in a boating accident. According to friends, he suffered a brief loss of consciousness at the scene. They report that he has a history of asthma. On admission, Mr Hayes was groggy but easily aroused, scoring a 13 on the Glasgow Coma Scale. He complained of blurred vision but his pupils were equal and reactive to light. Vital signs were stable. He presented with a 3.5 cm haematoma on his left, posterior temporal area and a deep laceration on his left forearm. A CT scan with contrast of the head and x-ray of the left forearm were normal. His laceration was sutured and he was given I.V. antibiotics via a cannula, as ordered. An indwelling urinary catheter was also inserted.

When you start your shift, you are assigned to Mr Hayes. The night shift nurse reports that Mr Hayes was admitted with a concussion. His Glasgow Coma Scale score is now 15, his speech is normal and his pupils are equal and reactive to light and accommodation. He received 1G of paracetamol for a headache at 6:10 a.m. His left forearm dressing is dry and intact.

As you are organising yourself to start your care, the charge nurse tells you that Mr Hayes' doctor has ordered removal of the indwelling urinary catheter and the I.V. cannula in preparation for discharge. You decide to proceed with your morning assessment and complete the discharge paperwork before checking and carrying out these orders.

Critical thinking exercise #1

Can you give three reasons why you might decide to keep the urinary catheter and cannula in place until just before discharge. They are:

1. _____

_____

2. _____

_____

3. _____

_____

Next you review the chart and jot notes in concept map form, while starting to fill in the discharge sheet you'll be giving to Mr Hayes.

Concept mapping exercise

Complete the concept map below, including the problem labels (titles for the various boxes), by integrating all of the assessment information you have so far on Mr Hayes. Note that information from the chart review is already added for you.

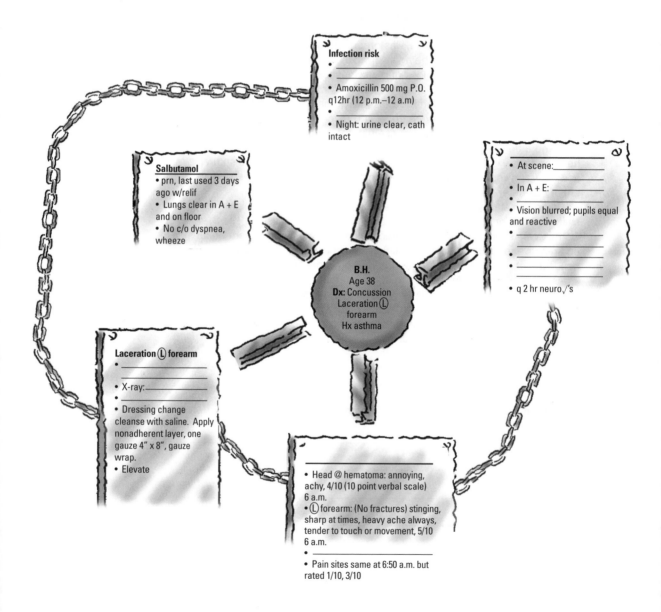

Infection risk
- _____
- Amoxicillin 500 mg P.O. q12hr (12 p.m.–12 a.m)
- Night: urine clear, cath intact

Salbutamol
- prn, last used 3 days ago w/relif
- Lungs clear in A + E and on floor
- No c/o dyspnea, wheeze

- At scene:_____
- In A + E: _____
- Vision blurred; pupils equal and reactive
- _____
- _____
- _____
- q 2 hr neuro√'s

B.H.
Age 38
Dx: Concussion
Laceration Ⓛ
forearm
Hx asthma

Laceration Ⓛ forearm
- _____
- X-ray: _____
- Dressing change cleanse with saline. Apply nonadherent layer, one gauze 4" x 8", gauze wrap.
- Elevate

- Head @ hematoma: annoying, achy, 4/10 (10 point verbal scale) 6 a.m.
- Ⓛ forearm: (No fractures) stinging, sharp at times, heavy ache always, tender to touch or movement, 5/10 6 a.m.
- _____
- Pain sites same at 6:50 a.m. but rated 1/10, 3/10

You return to Mr Hayes' room to finish your assessment and redress the laceration on his left forearm. He's sitting up in a chair and you notice that he's sleepy and his speech is slower and less clear than it had been. Nonetheless, he reports, 'I feel fine. I'm just waiting for breakfast.'

Critical thinking exercise #2

1. The difference in Mr Hayes' level of consciousness (LOC) may reflect:
   a. early morning hunger.
   b. beginning infection from the indwelling urinary catheter or arm wound.
   c. an increase in intracranial pressure (ICP).
   d. a normal variant in some individuals.
2. Your first action after seeing the change in Mr Hayes is to:
   a. call the phlebotomist to obtain a blood sample to send for a chemistry profile and complete blood count, while you obtain a urine sample for urinalysis with culture and sensitivity.
   b. take his vital signs; measure his pupils; check the remainder of his neurological signs and assist him into bed with the rails up.
   c. put up the bed rails, give him his call bell, tell him to stay in bed and then leave to find his primary nurse or your mentor to ask for assistance.
   d. apply oxygen and then call the doctor immediately and request a repeat CT of the brain or magnetic resonance imaging of the brain because of a probable subdural haematoma.

Answer key

Critical thinking exercise #1

1. If Mr Hayes' condition suddenly changed before discharge, an I.V. line might be needed for new medications.
2. If an untoward event occurs, the indwelling urinary catheter will be necessary to assess the patient's fluid balance.
3. You're responsible for fully assessing the patient so you can complete your portion of the discharge plan.

Concept mapping exercise

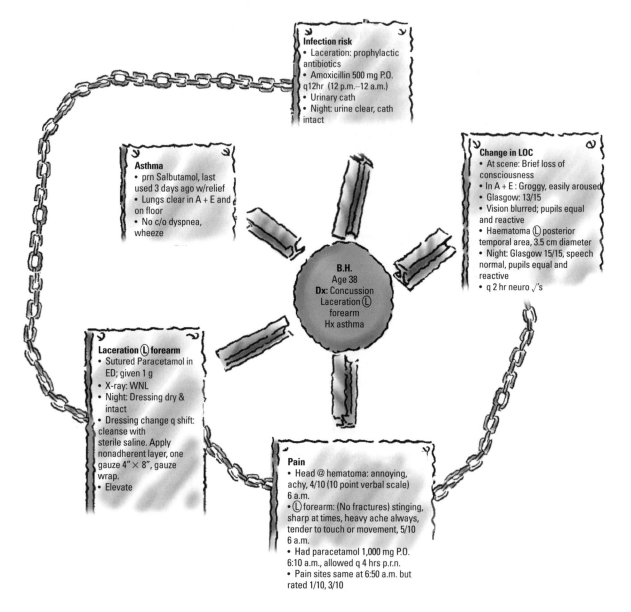

Infection risk
• Laceration: prophylactic antibiotics
• Amoxicillin 500 mg P.O. q12hr (12 p.m.–12 a.m.)
• Urinary cath
• Night: urine clear, cath intact

Asthma
• prn Salbutamol, last used 3 days ago w/relief
• Lungs clear in A + E and on floor
• No c/o dyspnea, wheeze

Change in LOC
• At scene: Brief loss of consciousness
• In A + E : Groggy, easily aroused
• Glasgow: 13/15
• Vision blurred; pupils equal and reactive
• Haematoma Ⓛ posterior temporal area, 3.5 cm diameter
• Night: Glasgow 15/15, speech normal, pupils equal and reactive
• q 2 hr neuro √'s

B.H.
Age 38
Dx: Concussion
Laceration Ⓛ
forearm
Hx asthma

Laceration Ⓛ forearm
• Sutured Paracetamol in ED; given 1 g
• X-ray: WNL
• Night: Dressing dry & intact
• Dressing change q shift: cleanse with sterile saline. Apply nonadherent layer, one gauze 4" × 8", gauze wrap.
• Elevate

Pain
• Head @ hematoma: annoying, achy, 4/10 (10 point verbal scale) 6 a.m.
• Ⓛ forearm: (No fractures) stinging, sharp at times, heavy ache always, tender to touch or movement, 5/10 6 a.m.
• Had paracetamol 1,000 mg P.O. 6:10 a.m., allowed q 4 hrs p.r.n.
• Pain sites same at 6:50 a.m. but rated 1/10, 3/10

Critical thinking exercise #2

1. C. A change in LOC is an early indicator of increased ICP. Hunger and early infection don't produce this sign. A subtle change in LOC is suspicious and may be the only early sign of increased ICP in a patient with a head injury. Pupillary changes are a later sign of increased ICP.

2. B. Because Mr Hayes isn't in acute distress, your first action would be to assist him to a safer position in case of further deterioration; then you would complete your neurological check and vital signs assessment so you can give objective, useful information to the primary nurse or your mentor. You should not have selected answer A because ordering laboratory work is usually out of the scope of practice of the nurse. Likewise answer C is wrong as making the patient safe is only a portion of your responsibility when a patient's status changes; a focussed assessment of the new findings must also be completed unless the change is severe and beyond your skill level. Finally answer D is also incorrect as there's no indication in the data given that the patient is in respiratory distress and may need immediate oxygen therapy. Independently calling a doctor for orders is usually outside the scope of practice for a student.

3 Nursing diagnosis and identification of problems

Just the facts

In this chapter, you'll learn:

♦ parts of a nursing diagnosis

♦ types of nursing diagnoses

♦ tips for identifying nursing diagnoses from concept map data.

A look at nursing diagnosis

Nursing diagnosis is the second step of the five-step nursing process. After you've assessed the patient and clustered the findings into related areas, you must analyse these clusters to identify the patient problems that nursing care can address. Next, you'll create specific labels—nursing diagnoses—for each of your patient's problems.

A definition for the diagnosis

A nursing diagnosis is a clinical judgement about a response to an actual or potential health problem or a change in circumstances, which provides the basis for the delivery of nursing care and the achievement of outcomes for which a nurse is accountable.

So what does this really mean? Let's break down this definition into digestible parts:

• A health problem is a circumstance such as illness, injury, or surgery or a lack of knowledge about a health issue. Examples of life processes include divorce, pregnancy or the death of a loved one.

- The problem must be responsive to evidence-based, clearly outlined interventions.
- The nursing diagnosis must reflect a problem for which the nurse:
  - is permitted to intervene
  - can be held accountable for the outcomes.

One, two, three …

To formulate nursing diagnoses, follow these three steps:

 Identify the patient's problems—using a concept map, if necessary.

Write a nursing diagnosis for each problem.

Validate the diagnosis.

Suppose your patient reports shortness of breath while walking short distances, your assessment reveals nasal flaring, a rapid respiratory rate and pursed-lip breathing. When clustering these data, you would see that these findings suggest a respiratory problem. Based on this, you would formulate an appropriate nursing diagnosis. Usually, your clustered data will lead you to establish several nursing diagnoses for each patient. You'll then arrange these diagnoses based on priority to ensure that you address the most crucial problems first.

Can't do without critical thinking

You'll need all your critical thinking skills to determine which nursing diagnoses are appropriate and to write diagnostic statements correctly. For example, understanding anatomy and physiology of the respiratory system and the way in which various lung disorders can alter respiratory function is critical to choosing between the nursing diagnoses *Impaired gas exchange*, *Ineffective airway clearance* and *Ineffective breathing pattern*. If you select an inappropriate diagnosis, you're likely to choose ineffective nursing interventions, and your care plan will not only reflect your lack of understanding but will also fail to help the patient.

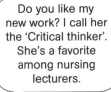

Do you like my new work? I call her the 'Critical thinker'. She's a favorite among nursing lecturers.

Parts of a nursing diagnosis

A nursing diagnosis is commonly referred to as a *diagnostic statement* or *identification of problem or need* because its format includes all the information that a nurse would need to quickly understand the factors affecting a particular patient and the specific symptoms of his problem. An experienced nurse who is pressed for time could, therefore, provide appropriate care for the patient without even reading the expected outcomes and interventions listed on the care plan.

Nursing diagnoses can have three parts:

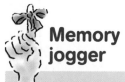

The first part is simply a **label**—for instance, *need for education*. It describes an actual or potential patient problem that nursing care can influence.

Part two is the **aetiology**, the related factors that precede, contribute to or are associated with the patient's problem. Examples of related factors include diseases, injuries, birth defects, inherited patterns, signs or symptoms, medical procedures, psychosocial factors, developmental phases, lifestyle and environmental factors. In the diagnosis, the aetiology should be preceded by the words 'related to', as in *Inability to maintain own hygiene needs related to weakness*.

The third part of a nursing diagnosis is a list of the **signs and symptoms** that support the diagnosis. This part is preceded by the phrase 'as evidenced by'. For example, a three-part diagnosis for a mental health patient might read *Ineffective role performance at work related to depression as evidenced by decreased concentration, and frequent crying while awake*.

When to use which parts

You may notice that nursing textbooks, journals and research papers sometimes refer to only one part of a nursing diagnosis (the diagnostic label) when defining patient problems. In some cases, the other two parts may be too specific for the discussion and are, therefore, unnecessary. In other cases, however, more detail is required and the diagnosis may include the aetiology as well.

The care plans that you write whilst practising should include at least the first two parts of the diagnostic statement, as this will enable you to develop your skills most effectively. Furthermore, if you're writing about a patient's existing problem, all three parts of the statement would be necessary for another nurse to understand the patient's situation. If the patient has the potential to develop a particular problem, but no current signs and symptoms, then the correctly written nursing diagnosis would contain just the first two parts of a diagnostic statement. Be aware that in clinical practice it might only be the nursing diagnosis or identified problem that is actually written on the care plan.

Types of nursing diagnoses

There are two types of nursing diagnosis:
- actual
- potential.

Actual diagnosis

An actual nursing diagnosis describes an existing problem—a human response (individual, family or community) to a health condition or life process that's validated by the presence of major defining signs and symptoms that cluster in patterns.

Everything's included

All three parts of a diagnostic statement are required for this type of diagnosis because:

- a label for the response or problem can be readily identified: *Ineffective infant feeding pattern* …
- the aetiology can be specified: *…related to cleft palate…*
- the patient exhibits qualifiable or quantifiable signs and symptoms of the response: … *as evidenced by the inability to form a mouth seal and abdominal distension from swallowed air.* (See *Adding evidence to the diagnosis.*)

Under construction

Adding evidence to the diagnosis

Writing a three-part nursing diagnosis is easy if you take it step by step. After writing the diagnostic label and the 'related to' portion of the nursing diagnosis, add defining characteristics—assessment findings that support the diagnostic label you've chosen. Precede these findings with the words 'as evidenced by'. Defining characteristics can be either subjective (such as the patient statement 'I feel dizzy') or objective (such as vital signs or physical findings).

For example

For an otherwise healthy patient with an open arm fracture, you collect the following assessment findings:

- vital signs—temperature 36.8°C, pulse 104 beats/minute, respirations 20 breaths/minute and blood pressure 124/76 mmHg
- displacement of the humerus of the left arm, above the elbow
- ragged-edged wound at the site of the injury with localised bruising, swelling and oozing
- displaced fracture of the left humerus on x-ray
- facial grimacing and tearfulness
- pain rating of 6 on a 0-to-10 scale
- constant twitching and movement of the legs
- tight gripping of the side rail by the right hand
- patient statement, 'I'm afraid of being put under for surgery. My aunt just died that way' (when told by the orthopaedic surgeon that open reduction and internal fixation of the fracture is the best treatment for this injury).

Given the patient's statement regarding surgery, one of the nursing diagnoses you should choose is *Anxiety;* you add the statement *related to fear of anaesthesia.* Then you should add the statement 'as evidenced by' and choose only those assessment findings most pertinent to this particular diagnosis. Your list should include enough information to validate your choice of diagnosis but need not include every large and small piece of evidence you collected. In this example, you would complete your three-part diagnosis with *as evidenced by body language and patient statement regarding anaesthesia for surgery.*

Potential diagnosis

A potential diagnosis describes a problem that the patient is at risk of developing. This type of diagnosis must:
• describe a problem or situation that could be prevented with proper planning and implementation of appropriate interventions
• be supported by risk factors (assessment findings) that make the patient more vulnerable to the particular problem.

Risky business

The diagnostic label for a risk diagnosis always begins with the words *Risk of* or *At risk of*. In addition, these diagnoses always contain only the first two parts of a diagnostic statement. Because the patient is just at risk of the problem, no signs and symptoms of the diagnosis are yet present; however, you will have identified the factors that suggest the patient is at risk and you're simply developing a plan to prevent the problem from occurring. Say, for example, your patient has a fractured femur, is restricted to bed rest and is obese. Based on these assessment findings, you might formulate a nursing diagnosis of *Risk of thrombolytic event or blood clot related to obesity, decreased mobility and bone fracture*.

> Risk diagnoses are easy to identify; they begin with the words 'Risk of'. Now that's risky business!

Creating nursing diagnoses from a concept map

If you used a concept map to plot out your patient's assessment data, as described in Chapter 2, you can then use that map to help you define the best nursing diagnoses for your patient.

Example

As an example, let's expand on the case scenario used in Chapter 2 (page 47). You've settled the child and his mother into a hospital room and orientated them to the call bell system and telephone usage. The patient's and his mother's responses to your questions help you realise that they don't know what's involved in getting ready for surgery, what to expect after the surgery or how long the surgery might last. The child is focused on his discomfort and points to the face labelled 8 on a 10-point faces pain rating card. He lies in the bed holding his abdomen, occasionally moaning, and complains of increasing nausea and head pounding. His skin is hot and dry, his colour is pale and he won't let you touch or listen to his abdomen. He hasn't experienced vomiting or diarrhoea so far, and his last bowel movement was yesterday. His blood pressure is 126/74 mmHg, temperature 38.5°C, pulse 120 beats/minute and respirations 28 breaths/minute. His lungs are clear and all his peripheral pulses are intact.

As per the doctor's prescription, and with the support and supervision of your mentor, you initiate an I.V. line and start infusing 0.9% sodium chloride solution. As you work, you explain to the patient and mother what you're doing and why. You also explain that the surgeon wants the patient to have a computed tomography (CT) scan of the abdomen before the procedure. You explain as simply as possible what a CT scan is. You also explain that the surgeon hasn't approved any pain medication because of the impending surgery (pain medication can mask important symptoms). When the patient is transported to the CT scan department, you provide more information to the mother on the surgical process and care after the procedure. The pharmacy sends up the ordered dose of I.V. antibiotics preoperatively and you verify with the mother that the child has no known allergies or sensitivities. You've already informed the surgeon of the mother's concerns about finances and obtained a referral for the social worker to visit. As per the mother's wishes, you've also notified the chaplain that she would like a visit as soon as possible.

With the above data in hand, you update your concept map, including the laboratory results that have returned. (See *Concept mapping for diagnosis*, page 60.)

Creating a problem list

When you develop a nursing diagnosis, you're translating the patient's history data, physical findings and laboratory data into a statement about his clinical status, responses to treatment and nursing care needs. A good way to start is to use the assessment information you've gathered to develop a problem list, which describes the patient's problems or needs. To help generate the list, you might want to use a conceptual model, such as Gordon's functional health patterns or a concept map.

Problem child

In the problem list, identify your patient's problems and needs with simple phrases, such as 'high fever' or 'gastrointestinal (GI) distress'. Then look at the assessment data categories, such as activity-exercise pattern or health maintenance pattern. For each category, determine if your patient is having a problem or is at risk of developing one. Then formulate a tentative nursing diagnosis for each problem or potential problem. (See *Problems, problems list*, page 61.)

Collaborative care

Not all nursing diagnoses can be managed solely by the nurse. To meet desired patient outcomes, some diagnoses require collaborative management by the nurse with a doctor, a nurse practitioner, a health care assistant, a pharmacist, a dietician, a social worker, a physiotherapist or another health care professional. This team of people is often referred to as the multidisciplinary or interprofessional team.

Concept mapping for diagnosis

Now that you have more information, you can update your concept map by adding all the assessment data you've collected (as shown here in colour) or just adding a few reminders based on the health assessment form you completed for admission.

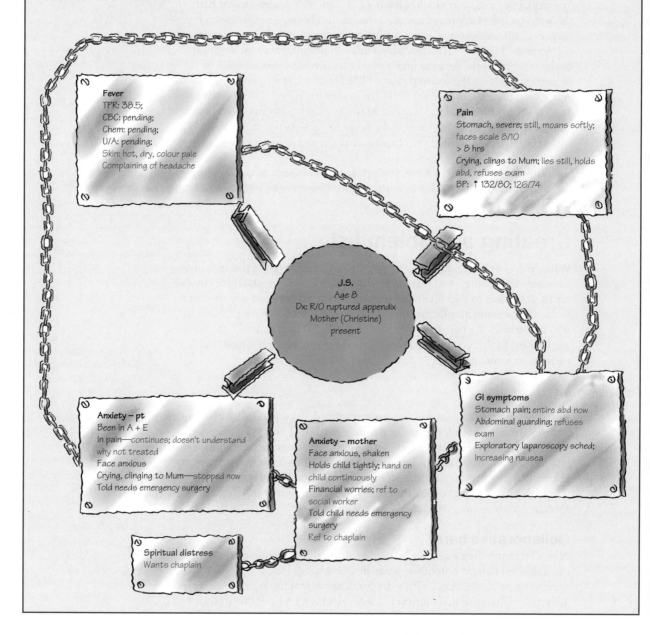

Fever
TPR: 38.5;
CBC: pending;
Chem: pending;
U/A: pending;
Skin: hot, dry, colour pale
Complaining of headache

Pain
Stomach, severe; still, moans softly; faces scale 8/10
> 8 hrs
Crying, clings to Mum; lies still, holds abd, refuses exam
BP: ↑ 132/80; 126/74

J.S.
Age 8
Dx: R/O ruptured appendix
Mother (Christine)
present

Anxiety – pt
Been in A + E
In pain—continues; doesn't understand why not treated
Face anxious
Crying, clinging to Mum—stopped now
Told needs emergency surgery

Anxiety – mother
Face anxious, shaken
Holds child tightly; hand on child continuously
Financial worries; ref to social worker
Told child needs emergency surgery
Ref to chaplain

GI symptoms
Stomach pain; entire abd now
Abdominal guarding; refuses exam
Exploratory laparoscopy sched; increasing nausea

Spiritual distress
Wants chaplain

Problems, problems list

Once all of your assessment data are updated on your concept map, you can analyse these data to create a problem list. Find a corner on the map and list the problems you've noted. Then begin to rough out the nursing diagnoses you believe might match those problems. For example, a problem list for the patient concept map at left might include the following problems and potential diagnoses.

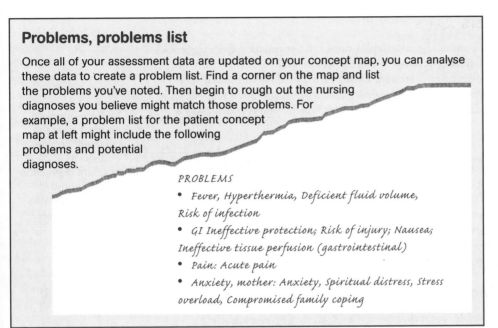

PROBLEMS
- Fever, Hyperthermia, Deficient fluid volume, Risk of infection
- GI Ineffective protection; Risk of injury; Nausea; Ineffective tissue perfusion (gastrointestinal)
- Pain: Acute pain
- Anxiety, mother: Anxiety, Spiritual distress, Stress overload, Compromised family coping

Under construction

The do's and don'ts of nursing diagnoses

Many nurses have trouble writing nursing diagnoses. Some find the language complex, abstract, vague, wordy or clinically not useful. The following do's and don'ts may help you to muddle through the mass of diagnoses to determine appropriate diagnoses for your patients.

Do

- Write diagnoses for problems that nurses are able to treat and that nursing interventions can resolve.
- List the diagnostic label first and the medical cause (aetiology) second.
- Make the diagnosis clear and precise.
- Include the diagnostic label, aetiology and signs and symptoms in all actual nursing diagnosis statements.
- Include only the diagnostic label and cause in all potential (*Risk of*) nursing diagnoses.

Don't

- Write a diagnosis that focuses on a medical problem. (Nurses should focus the delivery of their care on nursing problems.)
- Write a diagnosis that focuses on difficulty accomplishing a nursing intervention.
- Create a diagnosis for a treatment, diagnostic test or nursing task.
- Say the same thing twice.

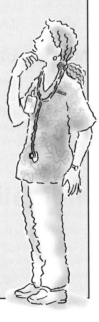

To complicate matters ...

However, not all physiological complications call for collaborative diagnoses. Suppose your patient is developing a break in the skin on their sacrum, or is at risk of developing an infection. In this case, the nurse can initiate and implement preventive measures or order definitive treatment. Thus, the problem is considered a nursing care issue for which a nursing diagnosis is appropriate.

Comparing nursing diagnoses and medical diagnoses

Once you become familiar with nursing diagnoses, you'll clearly see how nursing practice and medical practice differ. Both nurses and doctors identify patient problems, but they use different types of diagnoses and different treatment approaches.

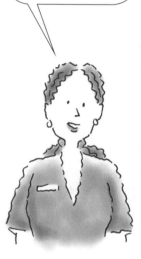

Remember, nurses treat the patient, not the disease. That important distinction is reflected in nursing diagnoses.

An interesting distinction

The main difference is that doctors are licensed to diagnose and treat a medical disease or condition, whereas nurses focus on diagnosing and treating a patient's *response* to a disease or condition. So a nursing diagnosis describes a *response* to a disease—not the disease itself.

However, nursing diagnoses aren't limited to patients' responses to diseases. Nurses also can diagnose the need for:
- patient education
- comfort and psychological support
- care until the patient is physically and emotionally capable of caring for themselves.

Another notable difference

Another way in which nursing diagnoses differ from medical diagnoses is that nursing diagnoses may change frequently during a patient's hospital stay or during the recovery process. As a patient progresses through the stages of illness toward problem resolution, the nursing diagnoses you formulate for him are likely to change correspondingly. (See *Adapting to changes*.)

Validating nursing diagnoses

After you have finished developing all of the patient's nursing diagnoses, you must go back and check each of the statements again to validate them. Start by determining the correctness of each diagnostic label, reviewing its definition and defining characteristics or risk factors and comparing them to the patient assessment data. Then critically analyse your information from

Adapting to changes

To illustrate the variability of nursing diagnoses versus the relative stability of medical diagnoses, consider the case of John, a 69-year-old retired carpenter with a medical history of hypertension and hyperlipidemia. He takes olmesartan and hydrochlorothiazide (Co-diovan) 80/12.5 mg and simvastatin (Zocor) 20 mg daily. He's married to 64-year-old Nancy, who works 40 to 50 hours/week and also is the primary housekeeper, cook and grocery shopper for the family. Follow his diagnoses through the course of an acute illness.

Course of the illness	Medical diagnoses	Nursing diagnoses
While his wife is at work, John develops sudden, severe weakness in his right (dominant) arm and right lower lip, with milder weakness in the right leg. He calls 999 but can't relay to the responders what happened or a medical or drug history. He's confused to time and place and says anxiously, 'I don't want to die.' He's taken to the hospital, where a computed tomography brain scan shows no signs of cerebral haemorrhage or clotting, but his blood pressure is 192/108 mmHg. John is admitted.	Rule out: • Stroke • Hypertension • Hyperlipidemia	• *Ineffective tissue perfusion (cerebral) related to hypertension and possible stroke* • *Risk of injury related to confusion and right-sided weakness* • *Fear related to sudden body changes and risk of death*
Nancy arrives at the hospital 5 hours later but stays for only 2 hours. Within these first few hours of admission John complains to the nurse about an inability to urinate. A bladder ultrasound shows 600 ml of urine in the bladder, and the nurse inserts an indwelling urinary catheter. John's urine culture is positive for infection, and antibiotic treatment is ordered. John's weakness and confusion don't worsen, and his lip drooping disappears. His blood pressure decreases to 186/96 mmHg. John still expresses fear that 'this is the end.'	Rule out: • Stroke • Hypertension • Hyperlipidemia • Urinary tract infection (UTI)	• *Ineffective tissue perfusion (cerebral) related to hypertension and possible stroke* • *Risk for injury related to confusion and right-sided weakness* • *Anxiety related to sudden body changes and risk of death* • *Urinary retention related to UTI*
Gradually, all of John's neurological symptoms disappear, except for some residual disorientation to time. John verbalises understanding that his condition is treatable. After 3 days, John and Nancy are informed that discharge is imminent, and the nurse assesses their ongoing care and learning needs. Nancy has visited John only briefly each day and states she has little time to learn a new diet; John says he can't remember it all. John is discharged from the hospital with a referral to the community health care team due to ongoing concerns for home safety and health maintenance and the need for more teaching regarding blood pressure management.	• Transient ischemic attack (TIA) • Hypertension • Hyperlipidemia • UTI	• *Lack of knowledge of medication regime related to new antihypertensive and anti-clotting medications prescribed* • *Lack of knowledge (patient and wife) of dietary needs related to new diet recommendations* • *Risk of injury related to possible recurrence of TIA or stroke*

(continued)

Adapting to changes (continued)

Course of the illness	Medical diagnoses	Nursing diagnoses
The district nurse visits John the following evening and completes an assessment. Nancy is present for the visit and expresses minimal willingness to learn about recommended dietary adjustments. She states: 'I'm just too busy; I can't do it all. He needs to do more for himself and the house. He doesn't seem to want to do anything at the moment.' John also admits to not taking his medications regularly before the hospital admission.	• TIA • Hypertension • Hyperlipidemia	• *Lack of knowledge (patient and wife) of dietary needs related to new diet recommendations* • *Lack of knowledge of medication regime related to new antihypertensive and anti-clotting medications* • *Altered family dynamics related to inter-spousal conflict over roles and skills* • *Risk of injury related to hospitalisation, hypertension, and risk of stroke or TIA*
During the course of John's care, the district nurse reports to the general practitioner (GP) that the patient shows difficulty with short-term memory and has a Mini-Mental Status Examination score of 26 (indicative of early dementia). The GP orders a magnetic resonance image of the brain, which shows signs of multiple small infarctions. Nancy verbalises more acceptance of John's care-giving needs and willingness to learn new skills when the testing shows he isn't deliberately refusing to be responsible.	• TIA • Hypertension • Hyperlipidemia • Multi-infarct dementia	• *Lack of knowledge (patient and wife) of multi-infarct dementia* • *Lack of knowledge (patient and wife) of dietary needs related to new diet recommendations* • *Impaired memory related to cerebral injury* • *Risk of injury related to hospitalisation, hypertension, and risk for stroke or TIA*

the assessment data and your knowledge of the associated medical disorders, verifying that you accurately listed the aetiology and stated the specific signs and symptoms that validate the diagnosis. This process of review and validation might help you find mistakes in interpretation of a definition or in placement of the parts of the statement.

Searching for support

If most of the patient's assessment data aren't consistent with or don't support the nursing diagnosis, you can either:
• reassess the patient for additional assessment data that *do* support the diagnosis
• revise the diagnosis so it's consistent with the assessment data.

Don't initiate the care plan until you've validated the diagnoses. If you write a care plan based on invalid nursing diagnoses, you'll waste time implementing it—and you could jeopardise your patient's well-being.

Prioritising nursing diagnoses

Usually, you won't have time to address all—or even most—of the nursing diagnoses you've formulated for your patient. You'll need to focus on the most important ones, which means that you'll have to be able to prioritise them. Then, when you plan your care, you address the highest-priority diagnoses first.

High, low and in-between

You can prioritise diagnoses into high-, intermediate- and low-priority:
- *High-priority* nursing diagnoses involve emergency or immediate physical care needs.
- *Intermediate-priority* diagnoses involve nonemergency needs.
- *Low-priority* diagnoses involve needs that appear less urgent; however this does not mean they are not important or can be ignored!

For example, for an acute-care patient in an adult setting, high-priority nursing diagnoses typically relate to airway, breathing and circulation (for example, *Decreased cardiac output related to cardiac tamponade*). Intermediate-priority diagnoses relate to problems whose resolution can impact the patient's speed or degree of recovery but aren't life-threatening (for example, *Risk of infection related to indwelling urinary catheter*). Lower-priority diagnoses commonly address anxiety, fear, self-esteem or a pre-existing chronic problem to which the patient has adapted (for example, *Insomnia related to variable shift work schedule as evidenced by sleeping during the day, and being awake at night since hospitalised*).

It is important to bear in mind that the patient is part of the prioritising process, and their perspective should also be considered. A nurse might consider risk of infection to be a higher priority need than responding to the patient's concerns about the impact of their illness on their employment, for example. However, from the patients' perspective their most pressing concern might be about the impact of illness on their employment, and the anxiety this creates could have a detrimental effect on the patient's recovery if this need is seen as low priority and not addressed.

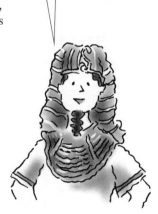

The pyramids have mystical powers. Maslow's has the power to help you prioritise nursing diagnoses.

Prioritising props

You can use the problem list you created to help you prioritise nursing diagnoses, or you can refer to Maslow's hierarchy of needs. This hierarchy classifies human needs based on the concept that physiological needs must be met before more abstract needs can be addressed. (See *The power of Maslow's pyramid*, page 66.)

Passing on the baton of care

You might not be able to solve all of the patient's problems and you may need to arrange a referral to another member of the interprofessional team who can help the patient to manage ongoing recovery or long-term impairment,

The power of Maslow's pyramid

Maslow's pyramid can help you prioritise a patient's nursing diagnoses. Physiological needs—represented by the base of the pyramid in the diagram below—must be met first.

Self-actualisation

Recognition and realisation of one's potential, growth, health and autonomy

Self-esteem

Sense of self-worth, self-respect, independence, dignity, privacy, self-reliance

Love and belonging

Affiliation, affection, intimacy, support, reassurance

Safety and security

Safety from physiological and psychological threat, protection, continuity, stability, lack of danger

Physiological needs

Oxygen, food, elimination, temperature control, sex, movement, rest, comfort

problems that a nurse in an acute care setting can't fully address. Likewise, if you are working in a long-term care setting your patient may develop an acute problem that requires referral to and the involvement of other members of the health care team on a temporary basis. Like in a relay race, the baton of care passes between members of the team to ensure all of the patients needs are met in the most appropriate way.

On the case

Case study background

Your patient, Harriet Zoose, has a medical diagnosis of *Acute exacerbation of ulcerative colitis*. When you obtain her health history, she tells you that she's currently experiencing painful abdominal cramps and has had very frequent bowel movements containing blood and pus for the past few days.

She rates her discomfort level at a 7 on a 10-point scale. She also states she has recently had trouble sleeping and feels extremely fatigued. She says the colitis has drastically decreased her sex drive, which is causing tension within her marriage.

On physical examination, you assess:

- hypotension
- low-grade fever
- reduced bowel sounds
- abdominal distension and tenderness
- pallor.

When you review her diagnostic data, you note that she has a moderately elevated white blood cell count; slightly elevated blood urea nitrogen (BUN) level; decreased haemoglobin level and total protein level; and a prolonged bleeding time. A gastroscopy performed the previous day found scarred and stenotic bowel segments, which are obstructing the intestinal flow.

Critical thinking exercise

Together, the nursing and medical diagnoses—and the care plan overall—should describe the complete nursing care the patient needs. For this patient, the care plan should include nursing diagnoses that address her *response* to her medical diagnoses. List four three-part nursing diagnoses for this patient. (Note that there are more than four correct answers.)

1. _____

_____

_____

2. _____

_____

_____

3. _____

_____

_____

4. _____

_____

_____

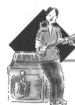

Answer key

Here are some examples of nursing diagnoses that could be appropriate for this patient:

1. *Risk of infection related to potential bowel perforation and general debilitation as evidenced by fever, abdominal distension and hypoactive bowel sounds.*
2. *Chronic pain related to abdominal cramping and distension as evidenced by pain scale rating and patient statements.*
3. *Insomnia related to anxiety and uncomfortable sensations as evidenced by patient statements.*
4. *Altered patterns of sexuality related to decreased physical energy and chronic, uncomfortable physical symptoms as evidenced by decreased sexual interest.*
5. *Dehydration related to acute diarrhoea and blood loss as evidenced by decreased haemoglobin level, increased BUN level and decreased blood pressure.*
6. *Fatigue related to decreased sleep, pain and exacerbation of colitis as evidenced by patient statements and decreased haemoglobin level.*
7. *Altered family dynamics related to increased symptoms of ulcerative colitis as evidenced by patient complaints of decreased libido and resultant marital tension.*

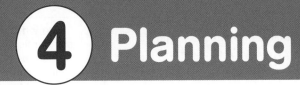

4 Planning

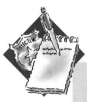

Just the facts

In this chapter, you'll learn:

♦ skills for developing and writing measurable, achievable patient outcomes or goals

♦ factors that influence behaviour and contribute to patient concordance

♦ guidelines for developing and writing effective nursing interventions

♦ the relevance of evidence-based practice in planning care.

Care plan components

After you establish and prioritise a patient's nursing diagnoses, you're ready to identify patient outcomes and develop a written care plan. Recall that the nursing care plan is a written plan of action designed to help you deliver quality patient care. It's based on the problems identified during the patient's admission interview and includes these three major components:
* nursing diagnoses
* expected outcomes
* nursing interventions.

One size doesn't always fit all

Care plans may be traditional (plans that are created from scratch) or standardised (pre-printed plans that can be tailored to a patient's individual needs). As a student, you'll most likely use some form of traditional care plan format until you've gained more experience in critical thinking. You may be instructed to use this care plan in

> Writing the care plan for a patient really starts with planning achievable goals with the patient and deciding the best ways to reach them. Gathering assessment data and developing nursing diagnoses form the basis for this plan.

conjunction with concept mapping. During your clinical placements, you'll consult the care plan tool used by the individual clinical area. Keep in mind that a patient's problems and needs can change, so you'll need to review the care plan often and modify it as necessary.

Take three giant steps

Writing an initial care plan involves these three steps:
- reviewing the assessed needs or problems and nursing diagnoses if needed
- identifying expected patient outcomes and specific nursing interventions to attain those outcomes
- documenting the nursing diagnoses, expected outcomes and nursing interventions in a clear, consistent format.

The first step above was covered in detail in the previous chapters. It's included here as a reminder that you should know your patient's established diagnoses and current status before you begin planning his specific care needs.

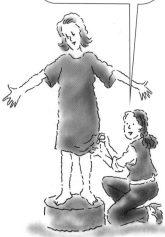

Tailoring a standardised care plan to each patient guarantees the best fit.

Identifying expected patient outcomes

During outcome identification, you must focus on determining appropriate goals, or expected outcomes, for a patient based on the nursing diagnoses you've already formulated for him. Remember, the ultimate goal of your nursing care is to help the patient reach his highest level of independence with minimal risk and problems by the time of discharge. If the patient can't recover completely, your care should help him to cope physically and emotionally with his impaired or declining health; the emphasis should be on quality of life.

Keeping it real

With these long-range goals in mind, you need to identify realistic and measurable outcomes and corresponding target dates for your patient. Expected outcomes are goals the patient should reach as a result of planned nursing interventions. Sometimes, a nursing diagnosis requires more than one expected outcome.

Outcomes are always geared toward the patient's performance—not the nurse's actions. An outcome can specify an improvement in the patient's ability to function— for example, an increase in the distance he can walk—or it can specify the correction of a problem such as a reduction in pain. In either case, each outcome calls for the maximum realistic improvement for a particular patient.

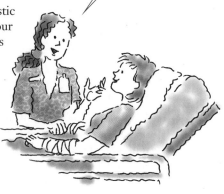

Make sure that the outcomes in your nursing care plan focus on the patient—not on actions you must perform.

The outcome statement

All outcomes must be patient-orientated and expressed in the form of a statement, called the *outcome statement* or *goal*. For instance, a patient with a nursing diagnosis of *Difficulty breathing and low oxygen saturations related to chest infection* might have an expected outcome of 'Show decreased difficulty breathing and increased oxygen saturation within 24 hours of intravenous antibiotic initiation.'

Parts of an outcome statement

An outcome statement consists of four components:

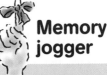

- a specific behaviour that shows the patient has reached his goal

- criteria for measuring that behaviour

- the conditions under which the behaviour should occur

- a time frame for when the behaviour should occur. (See *Understanding outcome statements*, page 72.)

Behaviour

A *behaviour* is generally defined as an action or response to stimulation that can be observed or heard. In terms of outcome identification, it's something (an action) you would expect to see or hear the patient do as a result of your nursing interventions.

Objectively speaking

Always begin your outcome statement with an action verb that focuses on a behaviour you can objectively observe and measure. Think of it as the thing that the patient will be able to do once the goal has been achieved. Examples of verbs that can be easily measured by sight or sound include:
- movements (for example, *mobilise, bathe, climb, give, move, perform, point, use*)
- speech (for example, *describe, express, report, state, verbalise*)
- other actions (for example, *arrange, avoid, demonstrate, exhibit, identify, maintain, modify, participate, seek, set*).
    If you could precede your sentence with *the patient will* then you have selected an appropriate verb.

Sounds subjective to me

Although it's important to consider the patient's thoughts and feelings when planning care, these can't be readily observed or measured. Avoid beginning an outcome statement with

I object to subjective outcome statements. Make sure that your nursing outcomes focus on behaviours that can be objectively observed or measured.

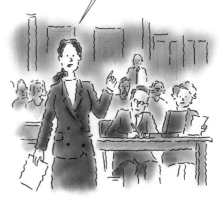

Understanding outcome statements

An outcome statement consists of four elements: behaviour, measure, condition and time frame.

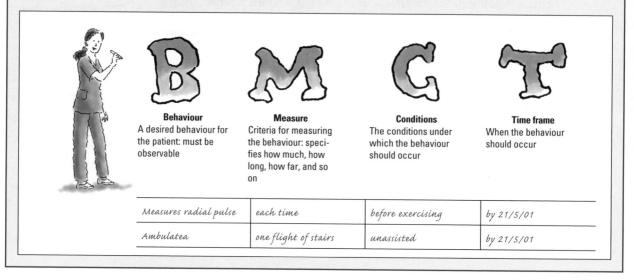

Behaviour	Measure	Conditions	Time frame
A desired behaviour for the patient: must be observable	Criteria for measuring the behaviour: specifies how much, how long, how far, and so on	The conditions under which the behaviour should occur	When the behaviour should occur
Measures radial pulse	each time	before exercising	by 21/5/01
Ambulatea	one flight of stairs	unassisted	by 21/5/01

a verb that's too subjective to evaluate, such as *accept, know, appreciate* or *understand*. After all, how can you objectively observe a patient's *appreciation?* Even when working with a mental health patient, you should try to write outcomes based on behaviours—not the thoughts or feelings that might be influencing the behaviours. For example, instead of including the outcome 'Patient will state that he feels less depressed,' you might include the outcome 'Patient's depression score will reduce by XX within seven days'; this outcome is a measurable improvement in a patient's mood.

Measure

Explaining precisely what's being measured and how it's being measured helps gauge your patient's progress toward achieving his goal. It also enables you and other team members to work within consistent parameters, ensuring the systematic evaluation of nursing interventions.

Specifics, please

Make sure your outcome statement indicates the criteria needed to measure the behaviour, such as:
- how much
- how long
- how far
- using what scale.

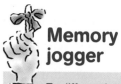

Memory jogger

To differentiate objective from subjective patient behaviour, think in terms of what you need to do to interpret it:

Objective—**O**bserve directly through sight or sound.

Subjective—**S**ense what the patient is thinking or feeling.

Conditions

Stipulate in the outcome statement, as necessary, the conditions under which the behaviour should occur. For instance, tell when during the day the behaviour should occur, how frequently it should occur and whether the patient requires any assistance in completing the action. For example, the outcome statement, 'Patient will drink 360 ml of clear fluids on day shift, 240 ml on evening shift and 120 ml on night shift,' gives more direction to staff and sets a clearer goal for the patient than the statement 'Patient will drink an adequate amount of fluid each day.'

Don't set the bar too high

Keep in mind your patient's overall condition, ability to perform the behaviour and agreement with the proposed target. Make sure the conditions can be realistically met.

For example, you're caring for a patient who has had an acute exacerbation of moderate chronic obstructive lung disease and now requires oxygen therapy for exertion and sleep. The patient's nursing diagnoses include *Lack of knowledge about measures to maintain maximum pulmonary function related to misconceptions about the disease process as evidenced by verbal statements regarding the disease* and *Activity intolerance related to disease process as evidenced by exertional dyspnoea.* You're aware that mild but regular exercise, such as performing self-bathing and grooming activities, can help the patient maintain his residual pulmonary function, so you establish an expected outcome of 'Bathe independently except for back and lower legs daily within 2 weeks.' However, this outcome may not be realistic unless the patient responds to your teaching plan for *Need for increased knowledge.* If the patient doesn't understand the basis for your outcome statement or doesn't agree that the goal is achievable, the expected outcome isn't realistic. In this situation, your outcome timing for the *Need for increased knowledge* diagnosis must be set before the target date on the bathing outcome, and you must be prepared to adjust the bathing outcome statement depending on the patient's response to the knowledge teaching plan.

Keep time in mind. Remember to include a time frame for completing each outcome.

Time frame

Although one of your primary responsibilities as a nurse is to help your patient achieve the highest level of independence or wellness before discharge, you need some way of monitoring his progress along the way. All patient outcomes must provide a realistic time frame for completing the desired behaviour. For example, in a care plan for a community patient you'll be seeing once a week, you might have a new outcome statement for each visit, as you assist the patient to learn to manage his disease process. At some point in his care, you may then be able to write a longer outcome target as he gradually integrates new information and techniques into his daily routine.

The long and short of goals

Long-term goals commonly require weeks or months to achieve. Short-term goals, on the other hand, take much less time to achieve; these are typically the goals (or outcomes) you'll initially address in your outcome statements. (See *Documenting long-term goals*.) The time frame for the goal is often linked to the health care setting. For example, in an acute ward the goals are likely to be short-term goals, whereas in the community or a care home the goals are likely to be achieved over a much longer peiod of time.

Writing outcome statements

When writing outcome statements, always start with a specific action verb that focuses on your patient's behaviour. By telling how your patient should look, walk, eat, turn, cough, speak or stand, for example, you give a clear picture of how to evaluate progress.

Documenting long-term goals

As a student, some of the expected outcomes you write will reflect short-term goals as your mentors encourage you to focus your care plans on outcomes that might be achievable by you during your time with a specific patient. However, you'll probably also be asked to get involved with discharge planning and this is where you may express some of the patient's long-term goals. Remember, planning for discharge should be a feature of the care that is planned and delivered throughout an episode of inpatient care, and not something that is left until the end of the patient stay in hospital. Some of the items you may be asked to consider when planning for discharge are:

- discharge outcomes—specify the outcomes expected by the time of discharge
- learning needs—list the topics that the patient and family should demonstrate an understanding of by discharge
- referrals—explain possible referrals needed to assist the patient and his family in reaching long-term optimum health outcomes
- documentation issues—identify the results of outcome evaluation that must be documented.

To each his own

Each clinical area or placement that you spend time in may have a different system of handling short-term and long-term outcomes in its care plans. Some examples are listed here:

- Acute care settings: Factors affecting discharge planning are documented on the initial assessment. The nursing care plan lists outcomes expected by discharge. Teaching flow sheets and discharge instruction sheets are used to document learning need outcomes and patient status and medical orders plus any referrals or follow-up care upon discharge. Patients are given a copy of their discharge instructions.
- Rehabilitative, home care, long-term care settings: The nursing or interdisciplinary care plan lists short-term and long-term goals for each diagnosis and specifies dates for re-evaluation of each. Discharge planning begins when the patient has been appropriately re-evaluated or requests discharge. Preparations for discharge are then listed as a goal on the updated care plan, as are any continuing care needs and referrals. A discharge summary is completed on the day of discharge and a copy is given to the patient.

Find out and follow the documentation procedures within each clinical placement and area.

Teacher knows best

Tips for keeping statements concise

These tips will help you write clear, precise outcome statements:

- **Avoid unnecessary words.** For example, with many documentation formats, you won't need to include the phrase 'The patient will …' with each expected outcome statement. In most cases, it's obvious that you're talking about the patient. However, you'll have to specify which person the goals refer to when family, friends or others are involved.
- **Only use accepted abbreviations.** It can be tempting to use abbreviations, but consider whether the abbreviation you use will be understandable and meaningful for every health care professional who utilises your care plan. Some abbreviations transcend specialities and professions, but others can become lost in translation!

Choose wisely

Be careful about your verb choice, though. Such verbs as 'allow', 'let' and 'enable' focus attention on your own and other health care team member's behaviour—not the patient's behaviour. In many cases, you can easily turn around outcome statements that focus on your behaviour so that they focus on the patient. For example, 'Medication brings chest pain relief' doesn't say anything about the patient's behaviour, but 'Expresses relief from chest pain within 5 minutes of receiving medication' does.

Include the nitty gritty

Also be sure to make your statements specific. For example, the statement 'Understands relaxation techniques' doesn't tell you much. (How do you observe a patient's understanding?) Instead, you should write, 'Practices progressive muscle relaxation techniques unassisted for 15 minutes daily by day 5 of hospitalisation.' This statement tells you exactly what to look for when assessing the patient's progress. Choose your words carefully and be clear and concise. (See *Tips for keeping statements concise*.)

For your consideration

When writing outcome statements, consider other members of the interprofessional team and the treatments they have prescribed or recommended. The outcome statements you write shouldn't ignore or contradict those orders. For example, before including the outcome statement, 'Mobilise 10 steps unassisted twice per day by postoperative day 3,' make sure that the physiotherapist hasn't recommended complete bedrest!

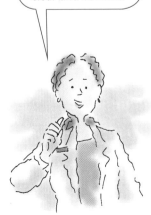

Although your outcome statements should be detailed, try to keep them clear and concise.

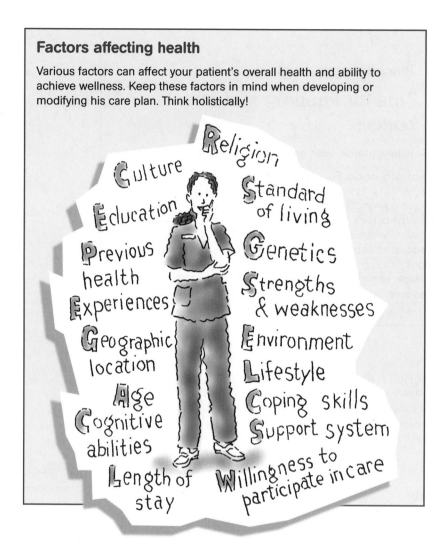

Factors affecting health

Various factors can affect your patient's overall health and ability to achieve wellness. Keep these factors in mind when developing or modifying his care plan. Think holistically!

Religion
Culture
Education
Standard of living
Previous health experiences
Genetics
Strengths & weaknesses
Geographic location
Environment
Lifestyle
Age
Coping skills
Cognitive abilities
Support system
Length of stay
Willingness to participate in care

Adapt the outcome to the specific circumstances. Consider such health-related factors as the patient's coping ability, age, education, cultural influences, family support, living conditions, socioeconomic status and anticipated length of stay. Also consider the health care setting. For example, the outcome statement, 'Mobilise outdoors with assistance for 20 minutes three times a day by admission day 5,' might be unrealistic in a hospital located within a large city. (See *Factors affecting health*.)

Patient participation

One way to help ensure the effectiveness of outcome statements or goals is to encourage the patient to participate in formulating them. A patient who helps write his outcome statements is more motivated to achieve his goals. His

Eliciting the patient's help

Discussing the care plan with the patient and keeping him informed about his progress and needed changes can be mutually beneficial. The patient remains informed and actively involved in health care decisions, and you elicit his concordance with achieving the outcomes stipulated in the care plan. Remember to keep the following points in mind:

- Discuss the care plan with the patient, and keep him informed whenever the plan changes.
- Assess the patient's knowledge about his condition or problem.
- Explain procedures and review laboratory findings.
- Respect the patient's wishes in the decision-making process.
- Begin discussing discharge plans at the earliest appropriate time, keeping the patient apprised of necessary changes to the plan.
- Seek the patient's permission to discuss his progress and needs with his family, particularly when planning ahead toward discharge.

Finding the right words in difficult situations

Some of the most difficult nursing diagnoses to work with are those that reflect the patient's perceptions and feelings. Let's look at and work through an example.

Example diagnosis 1

This diagnosis relates to how a patient perceives their health status: *Ineffective coping and feelings of denial denial related to new diagnosis of pulmonary hypertension (PH) as evidenced by patient statements, 'I feel better already. You just let me go home, and I'll get back to work in no time' and 'I think I was just working too much overtime and got exhausted. I just needed a break.'* The first tendency would be to write the outcome statement: 'Patient will accept his new diagnosis of PH by discharge.' However, because 'accept' is a subjective verb, this outcome is hard to measure. Taking one component at a time, let's see how to word a reasonable outcome for this patient:

- Objective desired **behaviours** might include 'Describes PH as the source of changes in health status and ability,' 'Expresses interest in learning more about the disease,' 'States understanding of the chronic and progressive nature of the disease' and 'Questions staff about how the disease may affect his ability to return to work after hospital discharge.'
- Let's assume that your interactions with the patient have led you to choose 'Describes PH as the source of changes in health status and ability' as an attainable behavioural outcome. Possible **measurement** of that behaviour might be 'by citing PH, not overwork or exhaustion, as the source of symptoms'.
- The **conditions** under which you might reasonably expect the patient to demonstrate this desired behaviour might be 'daily, when queried by nurse'.
- 'Within 3 days of diagnosis' is a clear **time frame** for the expected behaviour, although a specific date would be more helpful to other staff nurses.

input, along with family member input, can also help you set realistic goals. (See *Eliciting the patient's help*.)

Up for a challenge?

Not all outcome statements will be as straightforward to formulate as the examples previously presented. In such cases, remembering the four components and identifying each component separately can help you formulate outcome statements. (See *Finding the right words in difficult situations*.)

Developing nursing interventions

Once you've developed expected outcomes for a patient, it's time to start planning specific interventions to achieve them. As with patient outcomes, nursing interventions must be:
- realistic; they must be interventions that you actually have the scope to implement
- measurable; there must be a way of determining when the intervention has been implemented
- achievable within the time frame specified in the patient outcome.

Types of interventions

Interventions are grouped into two general categories:
- independent
- collaborative (or interdependent).

Independent interventions
An independent intervention is one that falls within the scope of nursing practice. It doesn't require a doctor's direction or supervision, so you can initiate the action on your own.

You're on your own

Many of the interventions you'll incorporate into the care plan are independent nursing interventions. They address aspects of care that you can do to promote change and facilitate wellness. These interventions cover such topics as:
- performing activities of daily living
- promoting safety and comfort
- patient education or health promotion.
    Independent interventions involve working directly with a patient, such as teaching him how to perform his own insulin injections. However, they also include the indirect activities you pursue to help him reach his goal, such as gathering resource materials about diabetes and insulin self-injection.

Collaborative interventions
A collaborative intervention is one that's based on instructions provided by a doctor or one that you'll do in consultation with another member of the health care team, such as a dietician, social worker or physiotherapist. Collaborative interventions fall outside the realm of nursing practice, meaning that you can't initiate them on your own. However nurses are still accountable for the implementation of the interventions, and as such should use their own professional knowledge and skills to make judgements about the suitability of the intervention, and should not be afraid to query interventions when uncertain.

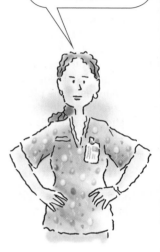

Independent interventions don't require any direction or supervision from a doctor.

Collaborative interventions are ones that you perform based on the instructions from another member of the health care team.

Hey, let's work together

Examples of collaborative interventions include:
- administering prescribed medications or fluids
- obtaining specimens for laboratory analysis

(See *Comparing independent and collaborative nursing interventions*, page 80.)

Writing nursing interventions

All nursing interventions are based on the goals stated in the patient outcomes and are intended to alter the aetiology, defining characteristics or risk factors for a specific nursing diagnosis. The number of interventions can vary for each outcome. What's most important is that the care plan is comprehensive enough to ensure that the patient can meet the outcomes. You'll usually list several interventions covering various aspects of care, all aimed at correcting the problem identified in the nursing diagnosis.

Each intervention you 'prescribe' must be written so that a caregiver (you or another nurse) has a clear picture of what to do to promote a positive change in the patient. The interventions should provide a set of directions, a 'map' that can be followed by whoever is delivering the care and implementing the interventions. (See *Tips for writing effective interventions*, page 81.)

Identify the activity

Keep in mind that all interventions are actions that *you* (not the patient) will do. Therefore, they should always begin with an action verb, for example:
- *Offer* fluids every 4 hours ....
- *Monitor* temperature, blood pressure and pulse ....
- *Assess* pedal pulses ....
- *Discuss* with patient how to perform regular breast examinations ....

Remember that the intervention should begin with an action verb, as in the examples above, and should contain enough information for any nurse (or appropriate member of the health care team) to be able to implement that intervention effectively.

Make it specific

Include as much information as is needed to know:
- how, when and where to do the activity
- how frequently it needs to be done
- special equipment needed
- additional instructions.

Watch the time

Remember that all of the interventions developed for a particular patient outcome must be achievable within the same time frame. This doesn't mean, however, that a particular intervention can't be used again to meet a new progressive outcome related to the original diagnosis.

Unlike outcomes, which are patient-focused, interventions focus on the actions that you, the nurse, will take.

Comparing independent and collaborative nursing interventions

Differentiating independent nursing interventions from collaborative interventions can be difficult. Some interventions can be classified as either independent or collaborative, depending on the wording used for the intervention and the nurse's understanding of her scope of practice. One way to differentiate is to consider whether the action is nurse prescribed or doctor prescribed.

This chart demonstrates a chain of related independent and collaborative nursing actions related to a practitioner order for bed rest.

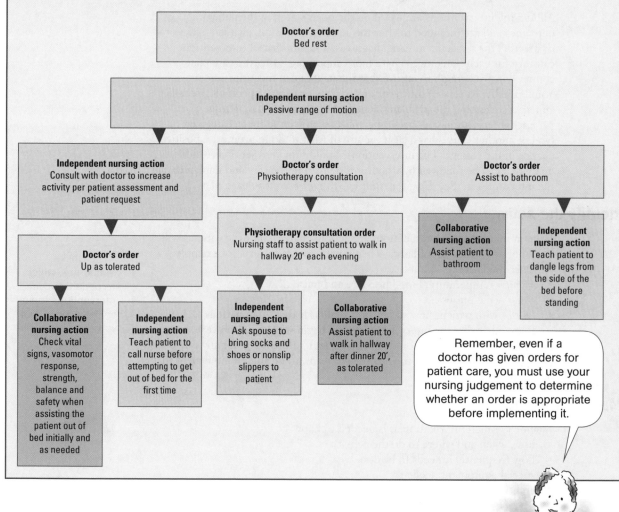

Teacher knows best

Tips for writing effective interventions

To write interventions clearly and correctly, follow these guidelines:

- Keep your interventions simple and to the point, and make sure they're aimed at helping your patient achieve the desired outcome.
- Clearly state the necessary action. Note how and when to perform the intervention, and include special instructions if necessary. For example, 'Promote comfort' doesn't tell you what specific action to take, but 'Administer prescribed analgesia 30 minutes before dressing change' specifies exactly what to do and when to do it.
- Make sure your interventions fit the patient. Consider the patient's age, condition, developmental level, environment and values. For instance, if the patient is a vegetarian, don't write an intervention that requires him to eat lean meat to gain extra pounds for healing.
- Keep the patient's safety in mind. Consider his physical and mental limitations. For instance, before teaching a patient how to self-administer medication, make sure he's physically able to do it and that he can remember and follow the regimen.
- Adhere to the policies and procedures in place in the clinical areas. For example, if the clinical area allows only nurses to administer medications, don't write an intervention calling for the patient to self-medicate.
- Consider other health care activities. Adjust your interventions when other activities interfere with them. For example, you might want your patient to get plenty of rest on a day when he has several diagnostic tests scheduled.
- Use available resources. If your patient needs to learn about his cardiac problem, use the resources in the clinical area, literature from the British Heart Foundation and local support groups. Write your intervention to reflect the use of these resources.

Keep in mind

When planning interventions, give some thought to:
- likelihood of success, taking into account the timing, interventions by other team members, amount of time required and cost factors
- resources available to you and your patient
- your ability to perform the intervention
- evidence-based practice
- the patient's ability and willingness to comply
- prior interventions that you or your patient have successfully used
- interventions from standardised care plans, nursing textbooks or nursing journals. (See *Plan to succeed*, page 82.)

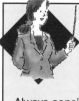

Teacher knows best

Plan to succeed

Always consider your intervention options carefully, and then weigh their potential for success. Determine if you can obtain the necessary equipment and resources. If not, take steps to get what you need or change the intervention accordingly. Also, observe the patient's willingness and functional ability to participate in the various interventions, and be prepared to postpone or modify them if necessary. For example, don't plan extensive verbal teaching with a patient who has significant hearing loss.

Using evidence-based practice

Evidence-based practice can be defined as the systematic and judicious use of the current best evidence to make decisions about patient care. When applied to nursing, the term *evidence-based practice* is used to describe the care that nurses provide based on research and identified standards.

Shifting sands

Because of the vast amount of available clinical research and accessibility to research findings, there has been a steady shift away from traditional, intuitive-orientated nursing toward evidence-based nursing. Nurses are following the growing trend among all health care fields of using well-designed and executed scientific studies to guide their clinical decision-making and clinical care. You should be aware of NICE guidelines, National Service Frameworks and other pieces of legislation and policy that will guide and influence the care you plan and deliver.

Putting evidence into practice

For your student care plans, your mentor may require you to write or explain your rationale for the interventions you've planned or completed. This rationale may also form part of your clinical assessments or the theoretical assignments you will have to produce and submit for assessment.

When planning care, you should use evidence-based research and your critical thinking skills to ascertain why certain actions or practices are being done. Asking pertinent questions can help you determine whether you're taking the right course of action and whether the interventions you've chosen will improve your patient's outcome.

Although tradition has its time and place, evidence-based practice ensures that nurses keep up with the times by using clinically sound best practices.

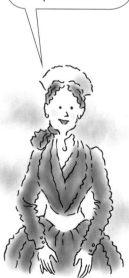

Don't be afraid to ask

Questions to ask yourself as you plan interventions include:
- Who determined the basis for this treatment?
- What's the rationale for this decision?
- What are the clinical ramifications of this practice?
- Is this the only way of doing this procedure?
- Could this be done more efficiently, or more cost-effectively?
- Is this the highest achievable outcome for my patient?

Evaluating sources of information

Truly evaluating the reliability and validity of the findings of a research study requires knowledge of statistics and research principles. However, keeping the following basic principles in mind can help you to identify valid sources of information that can be used to support evidence-based care—and avoid those that don't:
- Check resources for guidelines or standards of clinical practice related to your patient's medical diagnosis or the procedures or treatments he may be undergoing.
- Use resources written within the last 3 to 5 years, where possible.
- Use reputable, well-known journals and textbooks.
- Be wary of research that utilises small sample sizes because the conclusions from this research may be too narrow to generalise to a larger population.

On the case

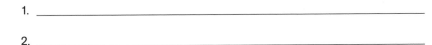

Case study background

You're caring for Johanna Keller, a patient with Parkinson's disease. After a recent medication adjustment, the patient's symptoms include mild, bilateral upper extremity tremors and slowed ability to initiate and sustain gross motor movements (such as rising from a bed or chair and walking). The patient is highly motivated to remain as active as possible for as long as possible. Based on her assessment data, you establish the following nursing diagnosis: *Impaired physical mobility related to Parkinson's disease as evidenced by upper extremity tremors and decreased ability to initiate and sustain gross motor movements.* You determine that an appropriate patient outcome is *Able to move purposefully in own environment independently or with mobility aids.*

Critical thinking exercise

Based on the diagnosis and outcome statement develop at least five nursing activities that would be appropriate for this patient.

1. _____

2. _____

3. _____

4. _____

5. _____

Out or in?

Read each statement. On the blank line provided, write 'O' if the statement is an outcome or write 'I' if it's an intervention.

_____ 1. Assist with mobilisation, as needed.

_____ 2. Demonstrate proper use of ambulation with quad cane within 4 days of discharge.

_____ 3. Administer oral analgesics three times per day, as prescribed.

_____ 4. Monitor vital signs every 4 hours until stable.

_____ 5. Offer sips of water and ice chips, as tolerated, followed by soft diet by day two postop.

_____ 6. Maintain acceptable body weight throughout length of stay.

_____ 7. Provide environmental cues (clock, calendar, pictures) to assist with orientation.

_____ 8. Encourage participation in daily self-care.

_____ 9. Avoid straining when having a bowel movement throughout hospitalisation.

_____ 10. Verbalise decreased pain as evidenced by lower score on pain-rating scale within one week.

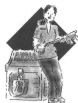

Answer key

Critical thinking exercise

1. Examples of nursing activities that would be appropriate for this patient include:
• Determine patient's readiness to engage in activity or exercise protocol.
• Collaborate with occupational and physiotherapists in developing and executing exercise program, as appropriate.
• Consult physiotherapists to determine optimal position for patient during exercise and number of repetitions for each movement pattern.
• Explain rationale for type of exercise and protocol to patient/family.
• Sequence daily care activities to enhance effects of specific exercise therapy.

• Re-evaluate need for assistive devices at regular intervals in collaboration with multidisciplinary team.
• Assist patient to develop exercise protocol for strength, endurance and flexibility.
• Incorporate activities of daily living (ADLs) into exercise protocol, if appropriate.
• Evaluate patient's progress toward enhancement/restoration of body movement and function.
Note that other nursing activities may also be appropriate.

Out or in? answers

1. Intervention
2. Outcome
3. Intervention
4. Intervention
5. Intervention
6. Outcome
7. Intervention
8. Intervention
9. Outcome
10. Outcome.

Just the facts

In this chapter, you'll learn:

♦ responsibilities associated with implementation of a care plan

♦ strategies for gathering and organising patient information

♦ methods for integrating care activities

♦ the importance of communicating with the interdisciplinary team

♦ two commonly used documentation methods.

Implementation overview

Once you've written a care plan—including the nursing diagnoses, patient outcomes and interventions needed to achieve those outcomes—you're ready to put the care plan into action.

Let's get hands-on

Implementation, the fourth step in the nursing process, is the step during which you'll have hands-on involvement with your patient. It encompasses:

- employing planned interventions
- using your critical-thinking skills to solve problems and set priorities
- continually reassessing the patient's response to your interventions
- communicating effectively with other members of the health care team
- documenting all of the care you provide.

All in a day's work

To implement a care plan, expect to perform some or all of the following types of interventions:

- carrying out routine assessment and monitoring of the patient
- delivering therapeutic interventions, such as administering medications or obtaining ordered specimens

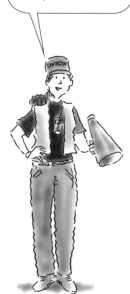

Less talk, more action. Implementation is the time to put your care plan into action.

- offering comfort measures
- providing nourishment
- helping with activities of daily living
- supporting respiratory and elimination functions
- providing skin care
- offering emotional support
- providing patient teaching and counselling
- communicating with other interdisciplinary team members.

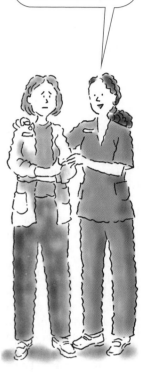

Don't be afraid to ask. If you need help, consult with other nursing staff before you perform an intervention.

Somebody point me in the right direction!

It's normal to feel slightly overwhelmed and even frightened when you begin implementing your nursing care plan, especially if you're a nursing student or are just beginning your nursing career. However, this lack of confidence will dissipate with time and ongoing experience. Remember, the care plan is a road map to helping your patient achieve wellness. It will point you in the direction toward achieving that goal, but it's your responsibility to determine if you need additional information or help from other staff before implementing an intervention.

Levels of responsibility

Your role in preparing and implementing a nursing care plan will vary with your level of nursing experience.

Student body

As a nursing student, your goal is to work from a care plan that you develop based on your assessment of the patient. In reality, you might not have access to your patient or their medical record until shortly before you become responsible for providing their care. In this situation, you need to review the care plan already in place as a blueprint for implementation. As you complete your own patient assessment, you become responsible for modifying the established care plan to reflect any changes and implementing your new interventions. The care plan you later write for your mentor may include diagnoses and interventions you actually had no time to initiate in the confines of your clinical time with the patient. (See *Who's the boss?*, page 88 and *The nursing shortage*, page 89.)

Following someone else's map

As a student and as a registered nurse, you may initially follow a care plan developed by another nurse, and you may not know much about the patient before you actually meet him and begin providing care. Your game plan remains the same, though—modify the care plan as needed as you develop

Who's the boss?

As a nursing student, you're likely to feel like you have too many masters. In the classroom and skills facilities, you must follow the directions of your lecturers. However, clinical placements can be much more confusing because you'll receive instruction from multiple members of the health care team. Understanding each person's role and practicing some basic skills can help you to work successfully with all team members in this challenging situation.

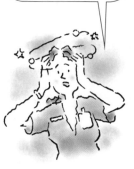

Do clinical placements have your head spinning? Take a minute to remind yourself what each person's role is.

Clinical placement staff

When you are in clinical placements the person who will be supporting you, supervising the care you deliver and ultimately assessing your competence, will be your mentor. All mentors must meet current professional body requirements, must have been prepared for their role and you should be spending a significant amount of your time with them. Your mentor is your guiding light! However, in addition to your mentor, you will also be responsible for frequent and open communication with the other nurses, midwives and members of the health care team who are delivering care. Remember, the staff nurse assigned to the patient bears overall responsibility for verifying that all required nursing actions are completed in a safe and timely manner, in accordance with the patient's care plan. The staff member assigned to the patient must know exactly which aspects of care you'll be providing, whether you might need supervision or assistance with a skill (in case your mentor isn't immediately available), and the results of your assessments and actions.

A learning experience

When you're on your clinical placements, you may feel that you waste a lot of time looking for the staff nurse or your mentor, leaving barely enough time to get your skills checked off and your work done. Use this frustrating situation to practice building some personal skills that will benefit you throughout your nursing practice, such as:

- flexibility—what else can you be looking up, cleaning up, finishing up, writing up or setting up while you wait?
- assertiveness—who else can answer your question or solve your patient's need, where else can you look for the information you need, how else can you correctly but politely convey the time frame or degree of urgency you're working under?
- coping ability—what else can you do to defuse your anxiety and frustration right now, how else can you think about this experience that will help you learn something useful about how nurses function day to day on the job, when else can you practice communicating honestly with a patient without off-loading your tension or anger onto him?

your own assessment data. As you're given new patients to admit to the area, you'll have opportunities to develop complete care plans for them.

Regardless of your place in the nursing hierarchy, it's up to you to learn as much as you can about your patient and their current condition before implementing care. You're even responsible for making sure that a doctor's orders are appropriate for a patient before you implement them.

Nursing shortages

One of the many ways financial constraints and the nursing shortage is affecting health care is the increasing shortage of staff members in many settings. However, this should not impact on the overall effectiveness of your experience, and you will find that Universities and clinical areas are adopting new ways of working to enable your learning experiences to be maximised.

Within the Universities

Within your University, the shortage may be reflected by reduced numbers of academic staff, and possibly an increase in the numbers of part time educators. However, this can actually be of benefit as you have access to an increased range of educators with experiences and insights to share. Many Universities also offer advice and guidance via student advisers, or student services, and your experiences in practice may be supported by roles such as the practice education facilitators or placement officers. The important thing is to make sure you are familiar with the support systems in place within your University and that you know who to go to if you have any concerns or queries.

In clinical areas

In the clinical setting, reductions in staff numbers, the shortening of admission times for acute care, the increase in care in the community, and rehabilitation patients being cared for in a variety of settings have all impacted on the ways in which care is managed and delivered. Advances in medical technology and knowledge have made minimally invasive surgical and diagnostic techniques with shorter recovery times much more common and increased the number of procedures that can be done in a short procedure unit. Each of these changes means that nurses have had to evolve new ways of working, and in order to maintain the learner's experiences Universities and clinical areas are working together to try out new models of clinical education. You may hear about or experience some of the following:

- Trainee mentors—Experienced mentors with demonstrated ability are partnered with less experienced nursing staff who are working towards their mentorship qualification. The student coordinates their clinical experiences with the trainee mentors work schedule; however, the experienced mentor also remains involved in the supervision and support of the learner, and remains accountable for assessment decisions.
- Joint student experiences—Junior- and senior-level students work together on a unit, with the senior students taking turns as team leader. This often happens when the senior students are in their final or management placement. Junior students perform interventions to their skill level and are supported by senior students. Whilst this is done under the supervision of a mentor it means that senior students obtain experience in delegation and management as well as senior-level skills and junior students are able to learn from other students who have understanding of and insight into their experiences.
- Alternative clinical settings—Students gain their clinical experience in a variety of health care settings that haven't traditionally been used for this purpose, such as independent sector environments, voluntary agencies, community support groups, occupational health clinics and prisons. Even international settings have been used in some Universities. Where possible a nurse or midwife should still take on the role of mentor, but where a nurse is not available within the health care setting (for example, in a day care facility staffed by social workers and care staff) long arm mentoring can be employed to ensure that the experience remains relevant and appropriate.

Getting started

Start your implementation of the care plan by assessing the patient's current situation. Then gather the supplies you'll need to complete the planned interventions.

Assessing the situation

Even if this is your first encounter with this patient, a great deal of information about the patient is available to you from various sources. For example, you can gather plenty of useful information by:

- listening to the handover of the departing nurse at the start of your shift
- reading the patient's chart, including information obtained during the initial history and physical examination
- talking with other staff, including your mentor and the patient's nurse
- talking with the patient and family members
- directly observing and assessing the patient
- reviewing laboratory and other test results.

Shifting gears and handing over

Begin your shift by attending handover and listening to the previous shift nurse's report about the patient. (See *Bedside handover—A new model*.) On a worksheet, write any pertinent information about the patient's vital signs, activities, intake and output, frequency of treatment and special instructions.

Take note of this

After listening to handover, you should review the patient's drug chart and care plan for any new instructions that may have been written. Note any changes in the patient's treatment or care regime on both the care plan and your worksheet. Also review the medication and I.V. fluid administration record, and make notes (on your worksheet) of the times that medications, I.V. fluids and other I.V. drugs are scheduled. Note the frequency of treatments, vital signs, dressing changes (and type) and blood glucose

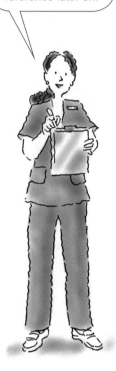

Write it down! The more information you write down, the more data you have to reference later on.

Weighing the evidence

Bedside handover—A new model

New research highlights the benefits of conducting the shift report at the patient's bedside. In addition to professional nurses, health care assistants can also attend the report. The research documents increase patients' satisfaction with their overall care, oncoming nurses' satisfaction with their information about patients' needs and status, physicians' satisfaction with the nurses' knowledge about their patients and management's satisfaction with the decreased amount of overtime required per shift.

However, where patients are being cared for in bays the maintenance of confidentiality can be an issue if bedside handovers are adopted.

Source: Anderson, C., and Mangino, R. 'Nurse Shift Report: Who Says You Can't Talk in Front of the Patient?' *Nursing Administration Quarterly* 30(2): 112–122, April–June 2006.

Electronic shift report

Whilst not yet widespread in the United Kingdom, some trusts are now utilising electronic patient record systems. Many electronic health record systems are programmed to send doctors' medical orders directly to the staff who will be implementing them. For example, new medication orders are sent to the pharmacy-specific section of the record system as well as to the nursing-specific section. Staff members in these departments can print out information they need to know from the records and use it to plan their work. Nurses usually obtain a printout (or electronic shift report) on each of their assigned patients at the start of their shifts. They might also regularly check the computer for new orders throughout their shift.

Although electronic shift reports are valuable, they shouldn't be used in place of verbal shift reports because the data they provide about a patient's current status are limited. For example, electronic reports don't tell you how your patient is doing, what issues are most important for follow-up or what the last assessment revealed. The electronic shift report printout is a good place to make notes about information obtained during the verbal shift report.

---

monitoring. This will help you to organise and integrate your planned independent nursing interventions with the collaborative interventions listed in the care plan.

Making contact

Next, assess the patient. Find where the patient is being cared for (side room or bay). Wash your hands, then go to the patient, introduce yourself and then check the patient's identification. Remember to use two patient identifiers, such as his name, birth date or hospital number. Whenever possible, ask the patient to tell you his name instead of calling him by his name.

Perform your initial assessment and make notes of your findings; these notes will provide the basis for your initial nurse's note in the patient's medical record. You can also use this opportunity to talk briefly with the patient (and any family members who may be present if the patient gives permission) and gather additional information about the patient's:

- perception of his current illness and his overall health and well-being
- ability to perform the interventions to meet the outcomes specified in the care plan
- available resources and support system.

Student report

If you're a student, provide a brief verbal report of your findings to the patient's assigned nurse and your mentor, alerting them immediately to any abnormal findings. Ask them to clarify anything you're unsure about or ask your mentor to check on the patient to verify your findings. (See *Nurses as resources*, page 92.)

Teacher knows best

Nurses as resources

Experienced nurses can be an invaluable resource. They've amassed a wealth of information through practical experience in providing bedside care. They can teach you organisational skills and strategies for thinking through situations that you may encounter in the clinical setting. Tapping into their knowledge can help you to fine-tune your assessment and care techniques in your quest to become a registered nurse.

Gathering supplies

After you've performed your initial assessment, you'll gather and assemble the appropriate equipment and supplies for other interventions you'll need to perform. Once you've properly prepared yourself and the necessary supplies, it's time to implement your care.

Providing care

Now you're ready to begin tackling specific interventions. Being prepared and developing a system that integrates various activities can help you manage your work effectively, whilst caring for the patient holistically and maximising the patients' involvement in their care.

Basic implementation steps

Although the specific care activities that you'll perform will depend on the patient's condition, some general practices apply to all patients. The timing of meals, therapies, tests and procedures the patient is scheduled to receive will determine which of the other interventions specified in the care plan you'll initiate next.

Meet Mr Med

When your patient is due to receive a medication, locate and prepare the medications under the supervision of your mentor or the patient's named nurse. (See *Safe drug administration guidelines*.) Follow a tried-and-true set of safeguards known as the 'five rights' to help you avoid the most basic and common medication errors. Each time you administer a medication, confirm that you have the:
• right drug
• right dose

I see medication administration in your future. Make sure that you have the right drug, dose, patient, time and route.

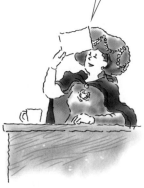

Teacher knows best

Safe drug administration guidelines

When administering a drug, be sure to adhere to best practices to avoid potential problems and manage those that do occur. You can help prevent drug errors by following these guidelines as well as trust policy.

Drug orders

- Don't rely on the pharmacy computer system to detect all unsafe prescriptions. Before you give a drug, understand the correct dosage, indications and adverse effects.
- Be aware of the drugs your patient takes regularly, and question any deviation from his regular routine. As with any drug, take your time and read the label carefully.
- Before you give drugs that are ordered in units, such as insulin and heparin, always check the prescriber's written order against the provided dose. Never abbreviate the word 'units'.
- To prevent an overdose from combined analgesics, note the amount of each analgesic in each preparation. Beware of substitutions by the pharmacy because the amount of paracetamol may vary.

Drug preparation and administration

- Always check the expiration date before administering a drug.
- If a familiar drug has an unfamiliar appearance, find out why. If the pharmacist cites a manufacturing change, ask him to double-check whether he has received verification from the manufacturer. Document the appearance discrepancy, your actions and the pharmacist's response in the patient record.
- Use two patient identifiers, such as the patient's name and hospital number, to identify the patient before administering any drug or treatment. Teach the patient to offer his identification bracelet for inspection when anyone arrives with drugs and to insist on having it replaced if it's removed. In the independent sector photo ID is often used instead of wristbands.

- Ask the patient to verify his allergy history before administering any medication.
- Ask the patient about his use of alternative therapies, including herbs, and record your findings in his medical record. Monitor the patient carefully and report unusual events. Ask the patient to keep a diary of all therapies he uses and to take the diary for review each time he visits a health care professional.

Avoiding common problems
Calculation errors

- Writing the milligrams per kilogram (mg/kg) or milligrams per meter squared (mg/m^2) dose and the calculated dose provides a safeguard against calculation errors. Whenever a prescriber provides the calculation, double-check it and document that the dose was verified.
- Don't assume that liquid drugs are less likely to cause harm than other forms. Paediatric and elderly patients commonly receive liquid drugs and may be especially sensitive to the effects of an inaccurate dose. If a unit-dose form isn't available, calculate carefully and double-check your math and the drug label.
- Read the label on every drug you prepare and never administer any drug that isn't labelled.

Incorrect administration route

- When a patient has multiple I.V. lines, label the distal end of each line.

Whenever administering any medications you must always follow the NMC Standards for Medicine Management (NMC 2007). These standards cover how to supply, dispense, store, transport and administer medications. The standards can be accessed directly from the NMC website.

- right patient
- right time
- right route.

Room service

At meal times, raise the head of the bed so that the patient can sit upright. Adjust their tray and assess their need for fresh water. Ask about any special requests, such as the desire for juice or other food items. Place the call bell within the patient's reach, and advise him to call you with any additional needs or concerns.

Before you leave

Each time you prepare to leave a patient's bedside or exit the patient's room, look over your care plan. Identify the interventions you've completed, and make note of any changes to the care plan that need to be made. Also note any changes in the patient's status; his response to treatment and care; and his refusal of care, treatments or regimes (all of which require nursing note entries in the patient's records).

Status report

Report any abnormal findings, patient or family concerns, changes in the patient's condition or uncertainty or concern about findings to your mentor and the patient's named nurse. Also report your completion of ordered treatments and regimens.

Integrating activities

Although you could approach each intervention separately when providing care, systematically checking off each intervention in the care plan, this approach isn't the most practical use of your time and energy. A more effective approach is to try completing as many interventions as possible during each visit to the patient. Coordinating and integrating your nursing care between or with activities of daily living, medication administration, vital signs assessments, treatments and other collaborative and interdependent care has several benefits:

- It saves time.
- It enhances your coordination skills.
- It allows you to provide efficient and timely care.

When taking an integrated approach, remember to review your care plan and notes carefully because you'll be attempting to complete several interventions during a single visit.

Implementation example

Because the care that you provide is specific to each patient, a sample scenario might help you to better understand ways in which you can successfully integrate routine activities to implement effective patient care. Suppose

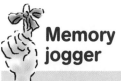

Memory jogger

Before you administer a drug, remember your nursing responsibilities for this intervention. To remember the sequence of the actions you must take, think 'Until Clear, Ask Many Times':

Understand the drug and how it works.

Clarify the drug order as needed.

Administer the drug.

Monitor the patient for therapeutic response to the drug and for adverse effects.

Teach the patient about the drug as needed.

you're working the morning shift (7 a.m. to 3 p.m.) in a hospital and you're assigned a patient with a neuromuscular impairment. After report, you review the care plan, which included the nursing diagnoses:

• *Inability to maintain activities of daily living related to neuromuscular impairment and generalised debility as evidenced by inability to wash body and obtain bath supplies.*

• *Risk of impaired skin integrity related to decreased mobility and poor nutritional intake.*

Your nursing care plan for this patient might look like the one shown in *Understanding implementation: Sample care plan*, pages 96 and 97.

Based on the care plan, interventions for this patient may include:
• taking vital signs
• administering prescribed morning medications
• assisting with personal hygiene (such as bathing, oral care, toileting and grooming)
• assessing skin, diet, fluid intake, musculoskeletal strength and mobility
• changing the bed linens
• positioning the patient
• providing a nutritious breakfast.

You'll also need to incorporate other assessments, such as assessment of cardiopulmonary status, bowel elimination and pain, into your care to gain a full picture of the patient's status.

Making the most of your time

Remember, to provide the most effective care possible, you may need to integrate several interventions. Here are some ways in which you can integrate the care-giving tasks that you need to perform:

• If the patient's ability allows, ask him to wash his face while you're setting up supplies for his bed bath. Observe the patient's reaction to this request and the action taken in response to assess the patient's interest in self-care, ability to understand and follow instructions, functional use and range of motion (ROM) of upper extremities and signs of discomfort.

• While supporting the patient to wash, ask about pain or discomfort with movement, level of fatigue, usual activity level before this hospitalisation, the availability of people to assist at home and any preferences for skin care.

• While helping the patient shave, assess endurance and fine motor skills and ROM of the hands and arms.

• When applying lotion to the patient's hands, assess bilateral grip strength, radial pulses, capillary refill and gross sensory disturbances.

• While washing the patient's lower extremities, assess strength and ROM of legs and feet, endurance, skin integrity, distal pulses, capillary refill, toenails and gross sensory disturbances.

• While helping the patient wash his perineal area, discuss bowel and bladder status or problems and observe skin integrity of the abdomen and groin.

• While assisting with oral hygiene, assess the teeth, gums, tongue and oral mucosa and encourage the patient to drink sufficient amounts of water. Teach the importance of adequate fluid intake to maintain healthy skin and bowel and bladder function.

Mealtimes are another good opportunity to assess your patient's status and their need.

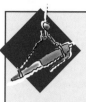

Under construction

Understanding implementation: Sample care plan

This sample care plan was developed for a patient who has problems with bathing and hygiene and who's at risk for skin breakdown because of his chronic illness and current hospitalisation.

Date	Nursing diagnosis	Patient outcomes	Interventions	Outcome evaluation (initials and date)
5/8/01	Self-care deficit (bathing and hygiene) related to neuromuscular impairment and generalised debility as evidenced by inability to wash body and obtain bath supplies	• The patient will wash his face, arms, frontal trunk, and perineal area on morning shift by discharge. • The family will demonstrate safe and effective assistance with patient's bath and hygiene on morning shift by discharge.	• Assess the patient's functional level every shift, and document findings. • Assist with or perform bathing daily while promoting patient independence in bathing the parts of his body within his reach and his maximal functional ability. • Change linens daily and as needed. • Assess the family's knowledge of proper bath and linen change procedures, safety measures, and rationale for personal hygiene in order to meet the patient's bathing and hygiene needs on discharge. • Instruct the family as needed on safe techniques for providing bathing and hygiene needs. • Observe family members demonstrate safe and effective assistance with the patient's personal care. • Assess the family's need for home care assistance to provide the patient's bathing and hygiene needs for safety or respite issues. • Refer the patient to social services, as needed, for assistance in obtaining home support services.	

REVIEW DATES		
Date	**Signature**	**Initials**
5/8/01	Jackie Miller, RN	JM

(continued)

Understanding implementation: Sample care plan (continued)

Date	Nursing diagnosis	Patient outcomes	Interventions	Outcome evaluation (initials and date)
5/8/01	Risk of impaired skin integrity related to decreased mobility and poor nutritional intake	• The patient will remain free from skin breakdown during the hospital stay. • The patient will maintain adequate food and fluid intake during the hospital stay. • The family will demonstrate proper use and understanding of home measures to prevent skin breakdown by discharge.	• Assess skin integrity every shift and as needed. • Assess dietary and fluid preferences on admission. • Assess dietary intake and fluid intake and output every shift. • Assess the family's knowledge of principles and practices of skin care and their need for specialized equipment to promote good care at home. • Keep skin and linens clean and dry, and keep linens wrinkle-free. • Turn and reposition the patient every 2 hours and as needed. • Apply lotion to dry skin areas after bathing, at bedtime, and as desired by the patient. • Provide foods and fluids of choice that are nutritionally appropriate for the patient's diet and medical regime. • Promote patient intake of at least 1 L of noncaffeinated liquids per day. • Teach the family as needed about skin care and observation techniques, position change requirements, and nutritional and fluid needs to prevent skin breakdown. • Observe the family demonstrate and verbalise understanding of all instructions given. • Refer the patient to a dietitian for protein and calorie evaluation, as needed. • Refer the patient to social services for assistance in obtaining special equipment in the home, as needed.	

REVIEW DATES

Date	Signature	Initials
5/8/01	Jackie Miller, RN	JM

Working with the interdisciplinary team

Nurses aren't the only health care professionals involved in patient care. As you implement care, you'll need to collaborate with an interdisciplinary team to meet the diverse needs of your patients.

Share and share alike

The focus of an interdisciplinary team is on the patient and patient outcomes. Each team member shares responsibility for achieving these outcomes. To provide more effective and comprehensive care, you need to understand each team member's role. (See *Meet the interdisciplinary team*.)

Meet the interdisciplinary team

Members of the interdisciplinary health care team—and their roles—include:

- doctors, nurse practitioners and consultant specialty physicians—who assess, monitor and provide treatment guidelines for the patient's medical conditions
- primary nurse, advanced practice or clinical nurse specialist and nurse-manager—who assess, monitor, teach and intervene to help the patient meet his expected outcomes by discharge
- registered dietician—who assesses and monitors nutritional needs
- social worker—who provides support and counselling to patients and their families and helps with financial difficulties
- occupational therapist—who assists the patient in performing activities of daily living, participating in recreation and working to the highest functional level
- physiotherapist—who assists the patient to improve or restore physical functioning and prevent deconditioning
- pastoral care specialist—who provides religious and spiritual support to patients and their families
- pharmacist—who reviews, prepares and dispenses the patient's medications; provides information and guidance in the preparation and administration of medications; and provides patient education (in an outpatient setting)
- discharge planner—who coordinates access to ongoing services after discharge, such as transfer to another facility, arrangement for medical equipment in the home or referral for home health services
- health care assistant—who supports nursing staff and assists in the delivery of the care required.

Independent sector care home, hospice or palliative care

In a care home, hospice or palliative care setting, the interdisciplinary team may also include:

- volunteer—who provides emotional and diversional support and respite to the patient and family
- bereavement counsellor—who supports and counsels the family for 1 year after the death of the patient
- activities organiser—who facilitates and delivers a balanced programme of activities aimed at meeting psychological and social needs of residents in care homes.

Important reminder

Don't forget the most important members of the team: the patient and his family. No interventions can occur and no goals can be met unless the patient permits the care and is committed to the outcome.

Passing notes is permitted

When you're reviewing the patient's chart, be sure to read the progress notes written by other members of the health care team. Those notes will provide you with important information about your patient.

If you have questions about the patient's condition or treatment, contact the appropriate team members for more information. For example, a pharmacist can tell you how to space medications to eliminate drug or food interactions, whereas a physiotherapist can provide you with written instructions on the patient's prescribed exercises.

> Remember, patient care is a team sport.

Play well with others

You'll also need to coordinate care with other team members. For example, medicating your postoperative patient before respiratory exercises helps the patient cough and deep breathe more effectively with the physiotherapist. When working with other team members, remember to use good communication skills. Above all, treat all team members with respect, and they'll respect you in turn!

Documenting interventions

Documentation is an important component of implementation. As previously mentioned, you should take notes after each intervention you perform, including the nature of the intervention, the time you performed it and the patient's response as well as interventions you performed based on the patient's response and the reasons you performed them. You should record interventions whenever you:
- deliver any planned care
- give emergency care
- observe and respond to changes in the patient's condition
- administer medications
- perform procedures or interventions
- remember as a student nurse all your entries should be counter-signed by your mentor or another trained nurse.

Tailor-fit to house style

Where do you document your interventions? That depends on the policy in each clinical area. You can document them on evaluation sheets, on a patient care flow sheet that integrates all nurses' notes for a 1-day period, on integrated or separate nurses' progress notes and on other specialised documentation forms (such as the medication administration record). The policies in place in each clinical area also dictate the style and format of the documentation.

Focused documentation

Your documentation should be patient-centred and outcome-orientated. Stating the patient's response to your nursing interventions helps to make your documentation patient-centred. Linking your interventions and responses to the nursing diagnoses and goal statements makes it outcome-oriented as well.

Documentation formats

Various types of nursing note formats are used in the clinical setting. They may be done by hand or in a computerised system. Two of the most commonly used formats for documenting interventions are discussed here.

PIE system

The problem–intervention–evaluation (PIE) system organises information according to patient problems and was devised to simplify the documentation process. This system requires you to keep a daily patient assessment flow sheet and to write structured progress notes.

Piecing PIE together

Each piece of PIE has its own purpose:
• The problem category is used to identify the nursing diagnosis requiring the interventions.
• The intervention category describes the actions you took and any assessment data related to the interventions.
• The evaluation section describes the results of your interventions and any additional information regarding attaining your outcomes.
(See *Using PIE documentation*, page 101.)

SOAP format

SOAP is an acronym for subjective data, objective data, assessment and planning. The SOAP system, which is used in problem-orientated documentation, allows all health care team members to record their findings using narrative progress notes. This system allows readers to readily distinguish between the subjective and objective data so the correct plan of care can be chosen, and you can show that your interventions addressed the patient's documented needs. It also specifies the follow-up care that's planned.

The dirt on SOAP

To use the SOAP format, document the following information for each problem:
• Subjective data: Information the patient or family members tell you, such as the chief complaint.

Using PIE documentation

For the nursing diagnosis *Inability to meet own personal hygiene needs*, you would document your care using the PIE format in this way:

P—Self-care deficit: Bathing and hygiene

I—Assisted pt. with bath; he was able to wash his own hands and upper chest slowly without discomfort. Pt. unable to lift arms above chest; muscle strength grade 3/6 upper and lower extremities. Remains on practitioner-ordered bed rest. Changed linens and repositioned pt. onto left side after applying oil-based lotion to skin.

E—Continues to require major assistance with personal care. Plan to assess the family's ability to meet the pt.'s bathing and hygiene needs when they visit in the afternoon.

For the nursing diagnosis *Risk of impaired skin integrity*, you would document your care using the PIE format in this way:

P—Risk of impaired skin integrity

I—Pt. assessment revealed warm, dry skin that's papery on the lower legs with some flaking. Sacral area is reddened from lying supine, but colour clears when the patient is repositioned onto left side. No other areas of redness or any other defects present. Radial, dorsalis pedis, and posterior tibial pulses +2 and equal bilaterally; all nail beds show brisk capillary refill. Applied lotion after bath. Pt. ate 50% of breakfast; states "I don't get too hungry anymore. I like a hot breakfast but I don't care for bacon or sausage, just eggs or oatmeal". Instructed pt. that dietitian can visit and help him choose meals he likes as well as find ways to keep up his protein and calories so his skin remains healthy. Pt. agreeable but requests visit in the afternoons, when his wife is here. Also taught pt. importance of drinking 4 to 6 cups of noncaffeinated fluids per day for skin, bowel, and bladder health and applying lotion to dry extremities, particularly the lower legs, at least twice daily.

E—Pt. verbalised understanding of all instructions but prefers to have wife hear information as well; pt. states "she keeps track of everything now." Pt. offers to ask her to rub lotion on his legs and arms during her afternoon visits. Referral made to dietitian.

• Objective data: Factual, measurable data you gather during assessment, such as vital signs and laboratory test results.

• Assessment data: Conclusions based on the collected subjective and objective data and formulated as patient problems and nursing diagnoses; these conclusions are dynamic, changing as more or different data become known.

• Plan: Your strategy for relieving the patient's problem, including both short- and long-term measures.

(See *Using SOAP notes*, page 102.)

Using SOAP notes

For the patient problem *Inability to meet own personal hygiene needs,* you would document your care using the SOAP format in this way:

> S—"I can't get to my bath supplies because my strength is gone. I can't even move myself."
>
> O—Pt. unable to lift arms above chest. Washed own hands and upper chest slowly. Muscle strength grade 3/6 upper and lower extremities. Pt. remains on bed rest.
>
> A—Self-care deficit: Bathing and hygiene
>
> P—Continue to provide for pt.'s bathing and hygiene needs. Assess and instruct family regarding alternate methods for meeting bathing and hygiene needs.

For the patient problem *Risk of impaired skin integrity,* you would document your care using the SOAP format in this way.

> S—"I'm feeling some pressure and pain in my lower back."
>
> O—Papery dry skin on the lower legs with some flaking; sacral area reddened from lying supine.
>
> A—Risk for impaired skin integrity
>
> P—Continue to change position frequently. Apply lotion to dry areas.

On the case

Case study background

For your first clinical placement on a medical-surgical unit, you're assigned to care for two patients. Your first patient is Shirley Trotter, a 75-year-old who was admitted yesterday with pneumonia and severe shortness of breath. Your second patient is Carl Conrad, a 46-year-old admitted 3 days ago for an abdominal cholecystectomy.

Critical thinking exercise

To help prepare for your clinical experience, place these steps in proper sequence by numbering them from 1 to 9:

_____ A. Assess Shirley Trotter.

_____ B. Document your care and the patients' responses to your interventions.

_____ C. Receive the shift report from your patients' previous nurse.

_____ D. Greet your patients, introduce yourself to them and verify their identities per protocol.

_____ E. Check in with your mentor and prepare the patients' morning medications, gathering any other supplies needed.

_____ F. Receive your patient allocation, research the medical diagnoses and existing care plans, and establish preliminary priorities of care.

_____ G. Assess Carl Conrad.

_____ H. Review medication and I.V. fluid administration records.

_____ I. Complete as many interventions as possible during each visit to each patient's room.

_____ J. Administer your patients' morning medications (under the supervision of your mentor).

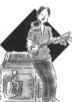

Answer key

Critical thinking exercise

1. F, 2. C, 3. H, 4. D, 5. A, 6. G, 7. E, 8. J, 9. I, 10. B

6 Evaluation

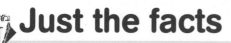

Just the facts

In this chapter, you'll learn:

♦ the importance of continually reassessing the patient's condition during all phases of care

♦ criteria for evaluating care

♦ the process for evaluating whether a care plan must be revised and the way in which revisions should be implemented.

A look at evaluation

Although designated as the fifth phase of the nursing process, evaluation is really an ongoing practice that occurs with every patient encounter. It encompasses:
- reassessing the patient
- comparing your findings with the outcome criteria or goals established in the care plan
- determining the extent of the patient's progress or outcome achievement (whether a goal was met, partially met or not met)
- writing evaluation statements
- revising the care plan, including nursing diagnoses, outcomes and interventions, as needed
- documenting your evaluation.

The value of evaluation

Each evaluation you make depends primarily on your ability to form an opinion or judgement about the data you collect. As a nurse, you'll use your evaluation findings to:
- determine if the original assessment findings still apply to the patient's condition
- uncover complications

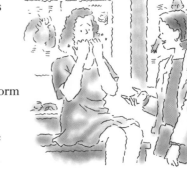

Don't be nervous about being evaluated. Evaluation is an ongoing and critical part of patient care.

- assess and analyse trends or patterns in the patient's response to all aspects of his care, including medications, changes in diet or activity, procedures, unusual incidents or problems and teaching
- determine how closely your care conforms to established standards
- assess the results of care provided by other health care team members
- identify opportunities to improve the quality of care.

Reassessing a patient

Reassessment is a necessary part of evaluation. After all, how else can you determine whether your patient's condition is improving, your interventions are working or your patient is making sufficient progress toward achieving his outcome goals?

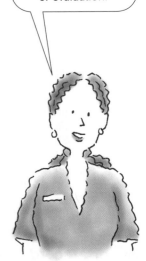

Reassessment is a necessary part of evaluation.

The patient and the process

It's important to note that reassessment includes not only periodically rechecking your patient's status throughout his care but also re-examining all phases of the nursing process in relation to the patient. This involves reviewing all the nursing diagnoses, patient outcomes and specific interventions written into the care plan. (See *Evaluation throughout the nursing process.*)

Evaluation throughout the nursing process

Assessment, or more correctly *reassessment*, takes place at all phases of the nursing process. Examples of the types of questions you can ask as you move through the stages of the nursing process are shown below. Remember that any change in the patient's condition that's outside of the expected findings requires you to notify the practitioner.

Nursing process step		Questions
Assessment		Have the patient's vital signs changed? What's the patient's current pain scale rating?
Nursing diagnosis		Is this diagnosis still realistic in the time allotted? Do the interventions still match the patient's expected outcomes?
Implementation		Did I observe a response when I implemented the interventions? Was the patient comfortable with the interventions?
Evaluation		How do the reassessment findings compare with the original findings? Can I document the nursing diagnostic goal as met?

Comparing patient data

In order to evaluate care, you must first compare your patient's prior assessment data to your follow-up assessment data to see whether their condition has changed. This comparison allows you to make inferences about the patient's condition and to alter the care plan accordingly.

Data déjàvu

When comparing data, remember to review all the patient's findings, including:
- their baseline level of functioning at the time of admission
- their most recent assessment findings
- any other pertinent data collected within the past 24 hours.

    Your comparison should include a careful review of the patient's functional level, vital signs and general overall status.

Begging the question

Next, you should compare the patient's current condition with his condition prior to the initiation of care to determine his response to your interventions (independent and collaborative). Ask yourself these two key questions:

 How is my patient responding to care?

What is their current condition (are they stable, improving or worsening)?

    Your answers to these questions will help guide your decisions about follow-up care. (For an example of how to evaluate patient data, see *Is my patient improving?*)

Report, record, react

The follow-up care you'll perform will be determined by the results of your reassessment evaluation. If the patient's condition is stable or improved, your next step is documentation of your findings. If, however, you feel the patient's condition is remaining static or deteriorating, be prepared to suggest alternative actions and give your rationales for them. Then proceed with further interventions as appropriate. Keep in mind that you'll need to document your findings and the care plan revisions. As a student nurse, you'll also need to report your assessment data to your mentor or the nurse in charge of the patient.

Evaluating interventions and goals

At some point, you'll need to conduct a systematic review of all your interventions to gauge your patient's progress toward achieving the expected outcomes. When you do this, you'll ask yourself many additional questions, such as:
- Do the reassessment findings show that the interventions are working?
- Are some interventions no longer necessary?
- Have any or all of the patient's short-term goals been met? Have long-term goals been met?

Is my patient improving?

You've been working with an elderly, bed-bound, terminally ill male patient. One of the major nursing considerations for this patient is his comfort level, which includes keeping him free from painful skin breakdown.

Initial assessment
The patient's initial assessment showed:

- very dry, flaking skin on the lower legs and feet
- build-up of dead skin on the soles
- deep-red heels that are continuously tender
- present and equal dorsalis pedis and posterior tibial pulses bilaterally
- absence of oedema
- sluggish capillary refill.

A nursing diagnosis of *Impaired skin integrity related to immobility, decreased nutrition and skin effects of aging* was identified on the patient's care plan, which also included the following expected outcomes:

- The skin on the patient's lower extremities will be pink, dry and intact by discharge.
- The patient's skin will be free from additional areas of impaired skin integrity throughout hospitalisation.

Your assessment
Your assessment on day 3 of admission reveals:

- soft skin on the lower legs and feet
- slight flaking of the skin on the ankles and feet
- decrease in residual dead skin build-up
- deep-red heels that are tender to touch
- unchanged pulses, oedema and capillary refill.

Comparing assessments
When you compare the new data you collected to the initial patient data, you determine that the patient's condition is improving and your plan is to continue to implement the nursing interventions identified on the care plan and to continue to monitor the patient. If your assessment had revealed that the patient's condition was unstable or worsening, in addition to continuing with established interventions you may also have added new interventions, such as consulting the doctor and tissue viability nurse for additional treatments or requesting a pressure-relieving mattress.

Complete or communicate

As a student, you might not be able to perform all of the interventions included in a patient's care plan. However, you're responsible for communicating to your mentor and the nurse in charge of the patient which interventions you did and did not complete. (See *Keeping track of interventions*, page 108.) This communication ensures that the nurse in charge knows what interventions still need to be completed so that the patient receives all of the planned nursing interventions.

Teacher knows best

Keeping track of interventions

One suggestion for keeping track of the interventions you perform is to check off the interventions after you perform them, and then write down data that suggest the patient is making progress toward achieving the goal. Also remember to evaluate and document in your notes how the patient tolerates the interventions you perform and any unexpected effects related to the intervention.

Achieving expected outcomes

On evaluation, you may determine, based on the patient's response to treatment and care, that the patient has met their short-term goals. For example, you may have successfully employed all of the interventions needed to return your patient's assessment findings to within normal limits. Hence, your evaluation would lead you to assume that the expected outcome has been met.

To help clarify this concept, consider a practical real-life example, such as buying a new pair of shoes. (See *The blue shoe blues*.)

When expected outcomes aren't met

Achieving expected outcomes indicates progress in your patient's care. However, suppose that you perform all of the interventions in the care plan and your patient's condition doesn't improve or, worse yet, their condition has deteriorated. These findings indicate that the expected outcomes haven't been achieved. So, what do you do? At this point, you must reassess the situation.

A case of intolerable interventions?

You're caring for a 78-year-old man with a nursing diagnosis of *Inability to maintain own elimination needs related to weakness as evidenced by loss of muscle mass due to aging.* This patient's expected outcome is that he will mobilise to the bathroom with assistance the third day after admission. You begin performing the following interventions, as mentioned in the care plan:
• Assess the patient's functional level and strength before getting him out of bed.
• Dangle the patient's feet at the side of the bed before assisting him to a standing position.
• Assist the patient out of bed to the bathroom when needed.
• Instruct the patient to call for assistance with toileting before an urgent need, and explain planned interventions to achieve the expected outcome.

As soon as you begin assisting the patient to sit on the side of the bed to dangle his legs, you hear him state that he feels dizzy. You immediately help him to lie back down in bed and take these vital signs: blood pressure

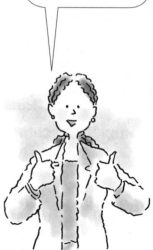

Positive outcomes indicate progress!

The blue shoe blues

Here's a practical example of how to evaluate whether expected outcomes have been met: Imagine that you've been invited to a graduation ball to celebrate the completion of your nurse training. You have a beautiful, new blue dress at home that you've been saving for just such an occasion. However, you assess your shoe wardrobe and are sad to discover that you have no blue shoes to match the dress. Your nursing diagnosis is *Lack of blue shoes*. Your short-term goal is to buy a new pair of blue shoes right away that are comfortable and reasonably priced. You remember that the shoe shop down the street is having a sale, and you drive there to search for shoes that are just the right colour, size and price. You make your purchase—a new pair of blue suede shoes—and drive home happy.

So, from a nursing perspective, how would you evaluate what you've just done? In this example, the best approach is to compare the diagnosis to the goal to determine what you've accomplished. The flowchart below takes you through this process step by step.

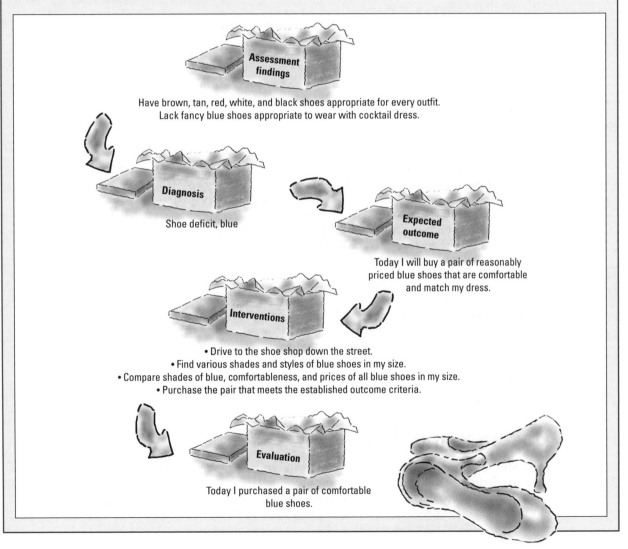

Assessment findings

Have brown, tan, red, white, and black shoes appropriate for every outfit.
Lack fancy blue shoes appropriate to wear with cocktail dress.

Diagnosis

Shoe deficit, blue

Expected outcome

Today I will buy a pair of reasonably priced blue shoes that are comfortable and match my dress.

Interventions

• Drive to the shoe shop down the street.
• Find various shades and styles of blue shoes in my size.
• Compare shades of blue, comfortableness, and prices of all blue shoes in my size.
• Purchase the pair that meets the established outcome criteria.

Evaluation

Today I purchased a pair of comfortable blue shoes.

80/58 mmHg, pulse 110 beats/minute and oxygen saturation per pulse oximetry 97% on room air. You check these measurements and find that the patient's morning vital signs were: blood pressure 110/64 mmHg, pulse 88 beats/minute and oxygen saturation per pulse oximetry 97% on room air. These vital sign changes and the patient's complaint of dizziness lead you to conclude that the patient's condition has changed. Given the circumstances, he's unable to carry out the intervention and, therefore, can't meet his expected outcome.

Reassess the patient's condition to determine whether the intervention you performed (assisting the patient to dangle his legs before standing) caused the response (dizziness, tachycardia and hypotension) or whether the response is a sign or symptom of a worsening condition or a complication. Ask yourself the following questions:

• Is this response a continuation or exacerbation of an existing problem or condition?
• Is this response due to something that has changed in the patient's condition?
• Is this a new problem that needs to be addressed by a revision of the care plan?

Subtle signs

During evaluation, always pay attention to even slight changes in assessment findings. Sometimes, a mild physiological adaptation, such as a response to a position change, can mimic a subtle change in condition. Because of a relative lack of clinical experience, student nurses commonly have difficulty making such distinctions, which can affect the care plans they create for patients. Remember, when you're in doubt, you and your patient will benefit most if you ask for help from another nurse or from your mentor.

The power of reassessment

When evaluation reveals changes in a patient's condition or expected outcomes that haven't been achieved by the nursing interventions set out in the care plan, or when your interventions create an unexpected patient response that leads to new symptoms or a worsening of the patient's condition, you must reassess not only the patient but also your expectations for the patient (expected outcome). In some cases, the care plan will need to be revised to reflect a different patient outcome and a new set of interventions.

Documenting changes

Remember to write a nurse's note (electronic or handwritten) that describes the patient's changed condition. Use the format preferred by the clinical area for this note. Also document any calls that you make to the doctor to inform him of changes in the patient's condition, including the time the call was made.

Writing evaluation statements

Part of the evaluation process involves writing a statement that describes whether the patient has achieved the expected outcome (short- or long-term goal) as it was written into the care plan.

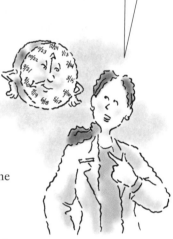

Short-term goals are those that can be accomplished during the patient's hospital stay, usually within a week.

Revisiting goals

As you may recall, short-term goals are those that can be accomplished during the patient's hospital stay (usually within 1 week or less), whereas long-term goals are those that can be accomplished over an extended time (usually more than 1 week).

May I opine?

Your evaluation statement should indicate whether the expected outcome was achieved. However, your documentation just prior to the evaluation statement should list the evidence supporting this conclusion. This evidence is the information you obtained in your reassessment and evaluation. These conclusions can state that an outcome has been fully met, partially met or not met.

Write right

In your actual patient notes, your evaluation should contain three types of information:
- results of your reassessment
- results of your comparison of the reassessment data with the patient's baseline data or normal findings
- evaluation statement that specifies the patient's status toward achieving his expected outcomes.

Evaluating short-term goals

Your evaluation of a short-term goal should occur within the time-frame established in the patient outcome statement. You should determine the patient's progress toward achieving the goal within the time-frame and revise the care plan if needed. Keep in mind that your patient may have more than one short-term goal for each nursing diagnosis.

Let's walk through it together

For example, if a patient outcome states that 'The patient will mobilise in the hallway two times with minimal assistance on the evening shift on 02/09/09,' you must evaluate the patient's progress toward accomplishing that goal by the end of your shift on that day. If for any reason the goal has not been achieved by the end of your shift, you must document this in your nursing notes in the form of an evaluation statement, such as 'Patient was unable to tolerate second attempt at ambulating in hallway with assistance; expected outcome not met.' Of course, your reassessment data supporting this evaluation would be documented in the chart according to the format used in the facility.

Evaluating long-term goals

Your patient's long-term goal may be the desired end-result of nursing care or, in some cases, a goal that extends beyond the usual time-frame of his hospital stay. Such conditions as stroke, myocardial infarction, traumatic brain injury, neurological or spinal injury, hip fracture and Alzheimer's disease commonly require long-term goals that extend over a continuum of care. Typically, patients with these conditions are discharged from the hospital to a continuing care facility or back home with a community care plan for continuing nursing treatment and care.

Long-term goals take more time to accomplish— sometimes weeks or months.

Taking the long road home

For example, the patient with a nursing diagnosis of *Inability to maintain own elimination needs related to weakness as evidenced by loss of muscle mass due to aging* may have the following expected outcome: 'Mobilise to bathroom with minimal assistance within 1 month after discharge to continuing care facility.'

Such a goal establishes a clear timeline for evaluating the outcome (within 1 month) and sets the criteria (with assistance, after discharge from the hospital or transfer to the rehabilitation centre).

Evaluating the care plan

In addition to periodically evaluating the patient's status and progress toward achieving outcomes, you'll also need to evaluate the care plan in its entirety. This means going through each section of the plan to determine whether the patient's problems have been resolved, outcomes have been achieved and interventions are still appropriate and current.

Re-evaluating the care plan is just as important as re-evaluating the patient.

Reviewing the plan

Your reassessment of the care plan will yield much information about what you and the patient have accomplished and what care still needs to be done. Ask yourself the following questions, taking each section in turn.

Look at the nursing diagnoses

• Does the patient still have the same problems (nursing diagnoses)? If so, has the focus of any of the problems changed in a way that would warrant rewriting the diagnosis?

- Were the diagnoses confirmed or ruled out?
- Does the patient have any new needs? If so, should any additional diagnoses be added to the care plan?
- Are all of the diagnoses prioritised?

Check patient outcomes

- Has the patient achieved the short- and long-term outcomes for each nursing diagnosis?
- Is each goal still valid and achievable within its given time-frame?
- Should the care plan include any additional criteria for achieving the outcomes?
- Does the patient agree with the stated outcomes?
- If the patient didn't achieve the outcomes, do you know why?

Review the interventions

- Do the interventions address the patient's specific needs?
- Are they achievable within the designated time-frames?
- Are they clearly written so that other team members can follow them?
- Should any interventions be discontinued or rewritten?

Evaluating the plan

Once you've reviewed the care plan, you can provide a written evaluation (on the care plan itself or in your progress notes) of each care plan section. Be sure to base your evaluation on information gathered from all sources, including your own observations and findings, the patient's medical record, the patient himself, the patient's family and other members of the health care team.

Record your evaluation using standard terminology that all team members can easily understand and follow. For example, use the following words:

- *Continue:* No change in diagnosis, patient outcomes or interventions is needed at this time, and the diagnosis hasn't yet been resolved.
- *Revised:* No change in diagnosis is needed, but the patient's expected outcomes and the associated interventions have been updated to reflect the patient's current status.
- *Discontinued:* A change in diagnosis is needed because additional data collection has shown that the diagnosis is no longer appropriate for the patient.
- *Achieved:* All expected outcomes have been met and the diagnosis is no longer appropriate for the patient, or one expected outcome has been met and, therefore, that portion of the care plan is marked 'achieved' while the other outcomes are ongoing.
- *Reinstate:* A previous diagnosis whose outcomes had all been achieved requires renewal because the problem has recurred.

Updating the care plan

In some cases, you'll need to make modifications to the patient's care plan as a result of your evaluation. Updating typically begins with determining whether the patient has achieved the outcomes. If the outcomes haven't been fully met but your assessment shows that the problem is resolved or was inappropriately identified, the plan can be discontinued. If the problem persists, continue the plan with new outcome target dates until the desired status is achieved. If the outcomes are partially met or unmet, identify interfering factors, such as misinterpreted information or a change in the patient's status, and revise the outcomes and interventions accordingly.

When plan A doesn't work . . .

Updating may involve:
• clarifying or amending the assessment to reflect new information
• re-examining and correcting nursing diagnoses
• establishing outcome criteria that reflect new information and new or amended nursing strategies
• adding the revised nursing care plan to the original document
• recording the rationale for the revision in the progress notes.

. . . go to plan B . . .

For instance, in the case of the patient who couldn't tolerate getting out of bed to use the bathroom, even with assistance, you could change the nursing diagnosis, patient outcome and interventions based on the inferences you made when comparing the baseline patient data with his reassessment findings. (See *Updating a care plan*.)

. . . or plan C

In the event that the patient can't tolerate the activities associated with sitting on the side of the bed and, therefore, can't meet the outcome goal, revise the care plan again, beginning with your reassessment. Other nursing diagnoses that can be established based on the given findings and reassessment data may include:
• *Dehydration*
• *Risk of injury*.

Keeping priorities straight

Be sure to reprioritise the nursing diagnoses when updating your care plan. This is especially important when the patient experiences unexpected changes in his condition or possible untoward reactions as a result of his treatment or care.

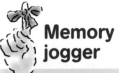

Memory jogger

If you know you need to revise your patient's care plan but can't remember where to start, think **REDO:**

• **R**eassess the patient.
• **E**valuate your findings.
• **D**ecide on a course of action.
• **O**rganise the care plan accordingly.

Updating a care plan

After your 78-year-old patient's experience with attempting to dangle and stand upright before walking into the bathroom, you re-evaluate the established care plan. After careful reassessment, you update his care plan to include an additional nursing diagnosis and expected outcomes. One possible update is presented below:

Date	Nursing diagnosis	Expected outcomes	Interventions	Outcome evaluation (initials and date)
4/1/01	Activity intolerance related to aging process and hypovolemia as evidenced by weakness, dizziness, and increased pulse rate during activity	The patient will tolerate sitting up at the side of the bed with assistance for 10 minutes, twice per day on 7–3 shift.	• Assess functional level every shift as needed. • Obtain positional vital signs, oxygen saturation level, and pain level before starting any activity and compare these findings to morning baseline data. • Assess patient intake and output over the last 24 hours. • Monitor for signs of fatigue and avoid activity during this period. • Maintain the patient's safety. • Raise the head of the bed incrementally to reduce dizziness. • Help the patient sit on the side of the bed with the assistance of two support personnel. • Remain with the patient the entire time he's sitting upright, and assess for changes in condition or activity intolerance. • Report significant changes in the patient's condition or activity intolerance to the doctor.	

REVIEW DATES

Date	Signature	Initials
4/1/01	Amanda Trotter	AT

When reprioritising diagnoses, ask yourself these questions:
- Will the patient's progress be hindered if the problem isn't managed now?
- Will the patient lose functional status if the problem isn't managed now?
- Will the patient be harmed in any way that will produce a detrimental outcome if the problem isn't managed now?

A new outcome

If you're changing the nursing diagnoses, follow through by updating the expected patient outcomes (remember to include realistic, measurable goals) and specific interventions needed to achieve them. Also, make sure your interventions address any new treatments or required care (independent or collaborative) resulting from the patient's changed condition.

Last but not least

Document all of your evaluations and, as a student nurse, communicate your findings to your mentor and the patient's named nurse. Be sure to follow the clinical area's procedure for recording nurses' notes and updating nursing care plans.

On the case

Case study background

You're assigned to care for Ella Racer, a 70-year-old admitted 3 days ago with dehydration. In reviewing the admission assessment data, you note that admission vital signs were: blood pressure 90/50 mmHg, heart rate 110 beats/minute and respiratory rate 18 breaths/minute. Her skin colour was pale and skin turgor was poor. Initial laboratory studies indicated an elevated serum sodium level and serum osmolarity. Her care plan includes the nursing diagnosis *Dehydration related to fluid loss through diarrhoea and inadequate nutritional intake.* Her expected outcomes are:
• The patient's fluid volume will return to normal and remain normal as evidenced by stable vital signs and a urine output at the volume established for the patient by day 3 of hospitalisation.
• The patient's electrolyte values will stay within a normal range by discharge.
• The patient will express and identify three ways to prevent dehydration by discharge.
   Nursing interventions for this patient include:
• Monitor and record vital signs every 2 hours.
• Measure and record intake and output every hour. Report a urine output less than 30 ml/hour.
• Administer fluids as ordered and monitor and record effectiveness of therapy.
• Administer antidiarrhoeal medication as ordered.
• Weigh the patient daily at 1800.
• Monitor electrolyte levels and report abnormal values.
• Explain reasons for fluid loss and teach the patient how to avoid further episodes.

Your reassessment on day 3 reveals the following vital signs: blood pressure 110/60 mmHg, heart rate 75 beats/minute and respiratory rate 16 breaths/minute. Urine output is greater than 30 ml/hour. Sodium chloride 0.9% with glucose 5% is infusing I.V. at 50 ml/hour. Skin colour is pink and skin turgor is normal. The patient has experienced no further episodes of diarrhoea and is tolerating oral fluids and solids. Electrolyte levels are within normal limits. The patient states, 'I don't know how I could prevent this from happening again.'

Critical thinking exercise

1. What reassessment findings show that the interventions are working?

_____

_____

_____

_____

_____

_____

2. Which interventions may no longer be necessary or could be altered?

_____

_____

_____

_____

_____

_____

3. Which of the patient's short-term goals hasn't been met?

_____

_____

_____

_____

_____

_____

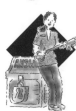

Answer key

Critical thinking exercise

1. Reassessment findings that show that interventions are working include vital signs that have returned to within normal limits (blood pressure 110/60 mmHg, heart rate 75 beats/minute and respiratory rate 16 breaths/minute); urine output greater than 30 ml/hour; normal skin turgor; oral fluid toleration and electrolyte levels within normal limits.

2. Because the patient is now stable, vital signs no longer need to be taken every 2 hours. Monitoring every 4 hours or 8 hours would be adequate. Urine output could also now be measured every 4–8 hours.

3. Because the patient stated 'I don't know how I could prevent this from happening again,' the goal of 'The patient will express and identify three ways to prevent dehydration by discharge' hasn't been met.

Just the facts

In this chapter, you'll learn:

♦ techniques for using traditional and standardised care plans

♦ the role of computers in generating care plans

♦ components of and uses for a critical care pathway

♦ types of care plans used in different health care settings.

Another look at the nursing care plan

By now, you're probably fairly well versed in the nursing process and its relationship to the nursing care plan. You know the five steps of the nursing process—assessment, nursing diagnosis, planning, implementation and evaluation—and understand that each step builds on the previous one and that all the steps interconnect, forming the basis of a care plan.

But how does it all come together? How do you gather all the necessary information about a patient and document it correctly? And where do you, as a nursing student, fit in?

> This chapter will help you put together the pieces of the care planning process.

Why you need a care plan

The nursing care plan is the core of your nursing practice—a vital source of information about your patient's problems, needs and goals and the quintessential blueprint to direct your treatment and care. When well-executed, this document can lead you step-by-step through your busy workday and help put your patient squarely on the road to wellness.

Flexible, but permanent record

There are a number of ways in which care planning links to the standards of conduct, performance and ethics for nurses and midwives (Nursing and Midwifery Council [NMC] 2008). *The requirement to keep clear and accurate records states that:*

- You must keep clear and accurate records of the discussions you have, the assessments you make, the treatment and medicines you give and how effective these have been.
- You must complete records as soon as possible after an event has occurred.
- You must not tamper with original records in any way.
- You must ensure any entries you make in someone's paper records are clearly and legibly signed, dated and timed.
- You must ensure any entries you make in someone's electronic records are clearly attributable to you.
- You must ensure all records are kept securely.

Effectively documenting care plans and showing that the stages of the nursing process have been followed can also demonstrate that these additional standards have been met:

- Treat people as individuals
- Respect people's confidentiality
- Collaborate with those in your care
- Ensure you gain consent
- Share information with your colleagues
- Work effectively as part of a team
- Manage risk
- Use the best available evidence
- Deal with problems

By nurses, but not just for nurses

Nursing is a unique patient-focused profession that's different from medicine and other health care fields, having its own set of diagnoses and outcomes and interventions that can be customised to meet each patient's needs. However, nurses don't work in a vacuum; they work in collaboration with other clinicians and staff to promote patient health and wellness. Consequently, although nursing care plans are developed by nurses, they may be used as a springboard to a plan that involves the entire interdisciplinary team, including:

- other nurses (clinical nurse specialists, registered nurses and nursing students)
- doctors
- occupational and physiotherapists
- speech and language therapists
- dieticians
- health care assistants
- social workers and discharge planners
- pharmacists
- clergy.

All on the same team

Each member of the interdisciplinary team may have some input in developing the care plan, but the registered nurse is responsible for making sure that it's carried out on a daily basis and documented according to the policies in place in that particular care setting. Other team members can also document their interventions on the care plan under their specified column or box. (See *The expanding world of care planning*.)

Students' role in care planning

As a student, you should read and be knowledgeable about your patient's care plan at the hospital, care home or community setting where you are on clinical placement. Each area and department operates differently, so it's your responsibility to become familiar with the system used.

RN recording rights

Keep in mind that registered nurses (RN) retain overall accountability for creating and updating a nursing care plan. This means the registered nurse remains the one who is accountable for the correctness, implementation and evaluation of the plan.

The expanding world of care planning

The nursing profession isn't the only profession concerned with demonstrating the unique and crucial nature of their skills in the health care setting. Like nurses, other health care providers are seeking ways to show that their actions reflect professional accountability and represent effective ways of delivering care.

Occupational and physiotherapists; speech and language therapists; and dieticians all assess patients, analyse their findings, develop treatment plans, implement their plans and reassess the effectiveness of their plans. The standards of practice for these professionals make it clear that these are mandated functions.

In many acute, continuing care and community settings these professionals are active members of an interdisciplinary team that develops an overall care plan for each patient. As such, a dietician might collaborate with nursing staff to include specific interventions in the nursing care plan that promote certain outcomes—for example, obtaining optimal nutrition or skin integrity. An occupational or physiotherapist might be involved in developing some of the nursing interventions for a patient with a diagnosis of *Impaired physical mobility*. Depending on the clinical area, these specialists may document their assessment findings and care on an interdisciplinary form or their own standard forms.

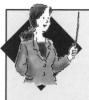

Teacher knows best

Paper trail

As you proceed through your clinical placements, the type of paperwork you're required to complete might change. An early focus may be on the nursing assessment and correlating those findings with the medical history and diagnosis. Later, you may be required to complete medication worksheets that focus on helping you learn about hundreds of drugs and what to teach the patients taking them. Finally come the nursing care plans themselves, in various formats and detail. All of these tools serve one essential purpose: to widen your knowledge base and sharpen your thinking skills so you can make decisions logically and quickly as you care for patients.

Student's right to write

As a student, you may use and follow the established care plan, and you will also be encouraged to create your own. After all, practice is the best way for you to learn! However, this should always be done under the guidance of your mentor, and all of your entries in patient documentation must be countersigned by either your mentor or another registered nurse.

Types of care plans

Care plans are usually written in one of two styles: traditional or standardised. Depending on the policies and practices in place in different clinical areas you may see both. There are various formats for standardised care plans; and in most cases, they are easier to use and more common than traditional plans. Another issue is the increasing use of electronic health records systems that include a care planning function. These systems are a variation on standardised care plans but require some special mention. Regardless of which type you use, your care plan should cover all aspects of nursing care, from admission to discharge.

Traditional care plans

Also called an *individually developed plan*, a traditional care plan is written to your patient's specific problems and causative factors. After you analyse your assessment data for a patient, you either write the plan by hand or enter it into a computer. (See *Traditional, but highly personalised.*)

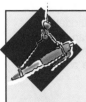

Under construction

Traditional, but highly personalised

Here's an example of a traditional care plan. It shows how these forms are typically organised. Remember that a traditional plan is written from scratch for each patient. These types of plans are becoming less common with the advent of electronic products containing modifiable standardised care plans.

Date	Nursing diagnosis	Expected outcomes	Interventions	Outcome evaluation (initials and date)
21/06/01	Ineffective breathing pattern R/T pain as evidenced by c/o pain with deep breaths or coughing and shallow respirations at 22 to 26 breaths/minute	The patient will maintain respiratory rate of 16 to 20 breaths/minute with normal depth while awake within 8 hours and ongoing.	• Assess and record respiratory status, including pulse oximetry q 4h. • Assess for pain q 3h and 1 hour after each dosage of pain medication. • Give prescribed pain medication as required • Assist patient to comfortable position q 2h while awake. • Demonstrate to patient how to splint chest while coughing.	
		The patient will rate pain as 3 or less on a 0-to-10 scale while using an incentive spirometer 10 times hourly while awake within 4 hours and ongoing.	• Provide rest periods between care activities. • Initiate oxygen therapy as ordered per given parameters.	

Nursing diagnoses, expected outcomes, interventions, and outcome evaluations are key elements of traditional care plans.

REVIEW DATES

Date	Signature	Initials
21/06/01	C. Planner, RN	CP

Home-baked from scratch

The basic form for the traditional care plan varies, depending on the function of this important document in your facility or department. Most forms have four main columns:

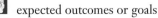 nursing diagnoses or identified problems

expected outcomes or goals

interventions

outcome evaluations

The form may also have columns for the date when you initiated the care plan, target dates for expected outcomes and the dates for review, revisions and resolutions. Most forms also have a place for you to sign or initial whenever you make an entry or revision.

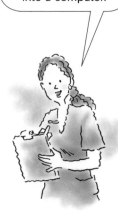

Traditional care plans can be written by hand or entered into a computer.

Looking towards an outcome

The information that you should include on a traditional care plan form varies, too. Because shorter hospital stays are more common today, in some clinical areas, you're expected to write only short-term outcomes that the patient can reach by the time he's discharged. However, other clinical areas—especially long-term care area—may also want you to plan long-term outcomes for the patient's maximum functioning level. These clinical areas commonly provide forms with separate spaces for short-term and long-term outcomes.

Personal, visual, clear

The traditional method has several advantages:
• It provides a personalised plan for each patient.
• The format allows health care team members and the patient to easily visualise the plan.
• Columns for outcome evaluations are clearly delineated.

Time isn't on its side

The main disadvantage of a traditional plan is that it's time-consuming to read and write because it requires lengthy documentation.

Standardised care plans

Standardised care plans are more commonly used. They eliminate the problems associated with traditional plans by using preprinted information. This saves documentation time. (See *Standardised saves time.*)

Standardised saves time

A standardised care plan can save you valuable time. The plan below is for a patient with a nursing diagnosis of *Impaired tissue integrity*. To customise this standardised care plan to one of your patients, you would complete the diagnosis—including signs and symptoms—and fill in the expected outcomes.

Date _15/04/01_

Nursing diagnosis
Impaired tissue integrity _Related to arterial insufficiency as evidenced by pain in calves and pressure area with walking; stage 2 ulcer on (R) fourth toe, bilateral +1 nonpitting oedema, cool temperature, and sluggish capillary circulation in right foot_

Target date

_11/04/01_

_11/04/01_

_11/04/01_

_19/04/01_

Expected outcomes
Attains relief from immediate symptoms: _Pain and oedema will resolve_
Voices intent to change tissue aggravating behavior: _Will stop smoking immediately_
Maintains collateral circulation: _Palpable peripheral pulses in lower extremities, extremities warm_
Voices intent to follow specific management routines after discharge: _Foot-care guidelines, exercise regimen as specified by physical therapist_

Date _15/04/01_

Interventions
• Provide foot and ulcer care. Administer and monitor treatments according to protocols.
• Encourage adherence to an exercise regime as tolerated.
• Educate the patient about risk factors and injury prevention measures. Refer the patient to a smoking cessation services on discharge.
• Maintain adequate hydration. Monitor fluid balance: _q8 hours_
• Elevate the head of bed: _6" to 8"_
• Additional interventions: _Inspect skin integrity q6h; assess peripheral pulses, skin temperature and color, and capillary refill q8h; administer analgesics before ulcer care and physical therapy as ordered p.r.n._

Date

_11/04/01_

_11/04/01_

_11/04/01_

_11/04/01_

Outcome evaluation
Attained relief of immediate symptoms: _Pain and oedema resolved, stage 2 ulcer continues; outcome partially met, extend expected outcome to 19/04/01 or discharge if earlier_
Voiced intent to change tissue aggravating behavior: _Hasn't smoked since admission, verbalises desire to remain nonsmoking after discharge with help of nicotine patch or gum if needed; outcome met_
Maintained collateral circulation: _Palpable peripheral pulses bilaterally, right diminished compared to left; right lower extremity cooler to touch than left; capillary refill sluggish but equal bilaterally; outcome partially met, extend expected outcome to 19/04/01 or discharge if earlier_
Voiced intent to follow specific management routines after discharge: _Verbalises understanding of foot-care and exercise guidelines given, and willingness to continue regime after discharge; outcome met_

Some standardised plans are classified by medical diagnoses or diagnosis-related groups (DRGs); others, by nursing diagnoses. The preprinted information included in a standardised care plan includes interventions for patients with similar diagnoses and, usually, generic outcome statements.

Insist on individuality

Early versions of standardised care plans didn't allow for differences in patients' needs. However, current versions require you to explain how you have individualised the plan for each patient by adding the following information:
- 'related to' statements and signs and symptoms for a nursing diagnosis—If the form provides a generic diagnosis, such as 'Acute pain related to _____,' you might fill in *inflammation, as exhibited by grimacing and other expressions of pain.*
- time limits for the outcomes—To a generic statement of the goal *Perform postural drainage without assistance*, you might add *for 15 minutes immediately upon awakening in the morning by 11/12.*
- frequency of interventions—To an intervention, such as *Perform passive range-of-motion exercises*, you might add *twice per day: in the morning and in the evening.*
- specific instruction for interventions—For the standard intervention *Elevate the patient's head*, you might specify *before sleep, on three pillows.*

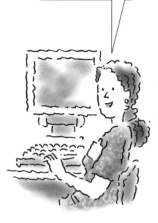

Standardised care plans are commonly completed on a computer.

Computers make combos less cumbersome

When a patient has more than one diagnosis, you must use all the standardised care plans, which can make records long and cumbersome. However, if your clinical area uses computerised standard care plans, you may be able to extract only the parts you need for each plan and then combine them to make one manageable plan. Some computer programs provide a checklist of interventions from which you can select to build your own plans.

Although standardised plans usually include only essential information, most provide space for you to write additional expected outcomes, interventions and outcome evaluations.

The pros

Standardised care plans offer many advantages because they:
- require far less writing than traditional plans
- are more legible
- are easier to duplicate

- make compliance with local policy easier for all members of the health care team, including experts, learners and support staff
- guide you in creating the plan and allow you the freedom to adapt it to your patient.

The cons (there's always at least one)

This method has one main drawback: If you simply check off items on a list or fill in the blanks, you might not individualise the patient's care or document your findings adequately.

Computerised care plans

Today, you're increasingly likely to encounter computerised care plans during your clinical placements.

Different strokes for different folks

Various types of software are available for different areas' needs. Some systems are programmed to generate a list of nursing diagnoses after the patient's assessment data is entered. You can modify the selected items as needed. Others require you to choose the diagnoses yourself from a master list. The system then adds these diagnoses to the patient's electronic health record (EHR).

EHRs also offer different styles of care planning. Some systems rely on generalised care plans written to a patient problem or profile, rather than to a specific nursing diagnosis. So, for example, a care plan entitled 'general care of the adult' could include nursing protocols for falls prevention and skin breakdown, as well as specific clinical guidelines for myocardial infarction.

RN input

Like traditional and standardised plans, a computerised care plan must be reviewed by a registered nurse at least every 24 hours. Remember that despite their efficiency and ability to access information quickly, computer software systems can't replace a nurse's critical-thinking and decision-making skills. Nurses still have to decide which diagnoses and interventions are most appropriate for any given patient and must evaluate when changes to the care plan are needed.

Care plans in different settings

As you begin your clinical placements, you'll notice that different units and care settings sometimes use different care plan formats. For example, acute care units, including mental health centres, commonly use standardised care plans, integrated or critical care pathways. Same-day surgery units often use a problem-list format rather than an actual care plan, but it serves the same purpose.

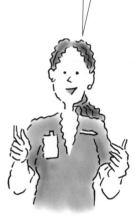

Note that different care settings use different types of care plans.

Have diagnosis, will travel

The standardised care plans available on each unit are usually selected to fit the type of patients common to the area. For example, a medical–surgical unit might have different standard plans than the maternity or psychiatric unit. However, a resource containing all plans should be available to all staff because patients may have more than one diagnosis, some of which may not be included in the standardised plans for the patient's assigned unit. For example, a patient on a psychiatric unit may have coexisting nursing diagnoses related to an ongoing medical diagnosis, such as diabetes or gastroesophageal reflux disease. Conversely, a patient with schizophrenia may be admitted to an oncology unit for treatment of cancer. Holistic patient care requires attention to all diagnoses because each impacts the patient's healing capacity.

Acute care hospital units

On most acute care units, care plans are separate documents that are formulated at the time of a patient's admission (typically within the first 8 hours). Although nursing interventions begin immediately with a patient's admission, the care plan takes careful planning and collaborative input and serves as a legal document of the care being given.

Most clinical areas require that care plans be reviewed and updated by a registered nurse at least every 24 hours, beginning with the time of admission. However it is usual to update care plans on every shift.

Fill in the blanks ...

Some units use preprinted plans on which the nursing diagnosis is already written; the nurse then makes the care plan specific to the patient. For example, for a patient with a nursing diagnosis of *Acute pain*, the nurse might fill in *related to surgical procedure* or *related to pneumonia with pleural effusion*, depending on the reason for the pain. The interventions, of course, would be filled in based on the patient's needs and circumstances.

... or check 'em off

Other units use preprinted care plans that include a comprehensive list of interventions. In this case, the nurse simply checks off the interventions applicable to her patient's problem.

Multiple problems

Usually, patients on medical–surgical units have multiple nursing diagnoses that must be addressed. All of the diagnoses for one patient are considered one care plan. For example, a patient admitted with a fractured left tibia might have the following diagnoses:
* *Acute pain related to compound fracture of tibia*
* *Risk of infection related to multiple breaks in skin integrity of left leg*
* *Impaired physical mobility related to fractured left tibia as evidenced by inability to bear weight on left leg and x-rays showing compound fracture.*

Keeping priorities straight

Within the care plan, the nursing diagnoses must be prioritised according to the level of importance for the patient. For example, suppose you've assessed a patient admitted with acute heart failure and have identified these diagnoses:
* *Excess fluid volume related to sodium and water retention*
* *Activity intolerance related to shortness of breath and fatigue*
* *Decreased cardiac output related to impaired contractility*
* *Impaired urinary elimination related to benign prostate enlargement*
* *Ineffective tissue perfusion (cardiopulmonary, peripheral) related to decreased cardiac output*
* *Anxiety related to acute increase in shortness of breath.*

You might prioritise these nursing diagnoses as follows:
* *Decreased cardiac output*
* *Excess fluid volume*
* *Ineffective tissue perfusion*
* *Anxiety*
* *Impaired urinary elimination*
* *Activity intolerance.*

Take the critical care pathway

A critical care pathway, sometimes known as an integrated care pathway, is a special type of care plan that's used by the interdisciplinary team, not just nurses, so it's more collaborative in nature. It includes assessment criteria, interventions, treatments and outcomes for specific conditions according to a time line that's based on an average patient's expected length of stay. Actual time-frames can be modified to meet each patient's needs.

Complete coverage

Think of an integrated or critical care pathway as a predetermined checklist describing the tasks you and the patient must accomplish. Unlike a nursing care plan, its focus is interdisciplinary, covering all of the patient's problems, not just those identified during a nursing assessment. For example, it may include specific interventions for physical assessment, investigations and procedures,

> Think of a critical pathway as a predetermined checklist that describes the steps you and the patient must take.

consultations, medication administration, nutrition, elimination, activity and therapy, patient education and discharge planning. (See the appendix for an example of an integrated care pathway.)

Day surgery unit

On a day surgery unit, nurses may follow an abbreviated standardised plan that addresses the patient's specific type of surgery or procedure. Additional medical diagnoses are listed and interventions are added related to those diagnoses if needed. The nurse typically reviews the problem list before and after the surgery or procedure. If the patient requires admittance to the hospital, a full nursing care plan is developed, using the problem list as a starting point.

Continuing care facilities

Care homes and other long-term care facilities often have their own systems for formulating care plans, and many develop their own paperwork and documentation. These systems are aimed at meeting the needs of their particular client group, and complying with the standards that regulate and govern the delivery of care in independent sector facilities.

Mirror, mirror on the wall

If you have a chance to do a clinical placement in a care home, you may find that this setting most closely mirrors the use of the nursing process and nursing and interdisciplinary care planning as you have been taught in the University. Because residents have chronic conditions requiring 24-hour care, nursing diagnoses may be relevant for long time periods. Expected outcomes tend to focus less on healing and resumption of prior function than on maintaining the present level of function and developing skills to adapt to limitations in function. However, always be alert for those situations where a rehabilitative goal is appropriate, such as fractured bones, episodic lung or urinary infections, situational depression or anxiety disorders, or new urinary incontinence issues.

Don't break the rules

Ideally, an individualised care plan for each new resident should be developed on the day of admission. However, it is likely that this will continue to evolve, particularly during the first few days, as the full scope of the patient's needs and problems are determined through ongoing assessment. Common nursing diagnoses in extended care facilities include:

- *Chronic pain*
- *Risk of injury*
- *Activity intolerance*
- *Risk of infection*
- *Risk of impaired skin integrity.*

Hospice care

Hospices also use care plans for their patients. In this setting, the care plan is prepared by an interdisciplinary team comprising nurses, health care assistants, physicians, therapists, clergy, volunteers, bereavement counsellors and social workers.

Creating care plans: A summary

As previously discussed, everything you do as a nurse focuses on the nursing process, and care plans are a natural extension of that process. Your patient's care plan is a summary of his problems, his goals, and the care he receives. It's also your key to helping him achieve wellness.

Revisiting the nursing process

You'll start developing your care plan beginning with your patient's initial assessment. This is when you'll talk with the patient and his family members to gather subjective and objective data, perform a physical examination and obtain the medical history.

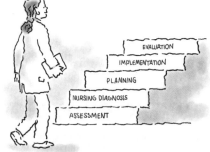

Taking it step by step

From all this information, you'll develop your nursing diagnoses, collaborate with the patient to identify his outcome goals and begin planning interventions to achieve those goals. The plan you come up with—the nursing care plan—directs your patient care from that moment forward.

Why you do what you do

As a student, remember to include a rationale (reason) and cite the reference source, as appropriate, for each intervention. The rationale is the 'why' behind the 'what'.

Why is it necessary to mobilise a surgical patient on the first postoperative day? Why should you assess lung sounds every 4 hours if your patient has heart failure? Right now, you're learning the answers to these and other questions in your classroom setting and by researching journals and other textbooks. With each new patient, you'll acquire more and more knowledge and hone your critical-thinking skills. Soon such questions, and their corresponding rationales, will become second nature to you.

As a practicing nurse, you won't include rationales in the patient's care plan. But don't think this lets you off the hook! Nursing is continually evolving, just like medicine in general. Long-trusted techniques and standards of care may be rejected as research shows better ways to accomplish the same tasks. Throughout your career, you'll need to stay up-to-date with the latest evidence-based practice and standards of care. In fact, the Nursing and Midwifery Council (NMC) requires you to engage in lifelong learning and fulfil their ongoing requirements to be eligible for re-registration.

Evaluating and reassessing at every turn

Keep in mind that, as you perform each intervention, you'll need to evaluate your patient's condition and response to the intervention. In some cases, these responses will require you to change the care plan accordingly. For example, your patient may not be able to walk the distance specified in his care plan or his pneumonia may be clearing up and you won't need to assess his breath sounds as frequently as specified in the care plan. Such changes mean re-examining the interventions and expected outcome and making necessary modifications if the patient hasn't yet achieved his outcome goal.

Sample care plans and concept maps

During your clinical placements, you'll probably care for patients in maternity, paediatric, psychiatric and medical–surgical settings. On the pages that follow, you'll find sample patient scenarios, with corresponding concept maps and care plans, for some of these settings. These care plans and concept maps are included to help you analyse how a care plan comes together. As you review these sample plans, try to think of other possible diagnoses, outcomes and interventions that might be appropriate for these patients.

Feeling the blues

A 65-year-old female, Julie Blue, is admitted with depression and inadequate nutrition due to lack of eating. Her husband of 45 years passed away unexpectedly 1 year ago, and she hasn't been coping well with his death. Her daughter brought her to the hospital because she couldn't get her mother to eat, bathe, get out of bed or brush her hair for the past 2 weeks.

The patient states, 'I just can't go on without my husband. He did everything.' The daughter also tells the nurse that the electric and water have been turned off because her mother keeps forgetting to pay the bills.

The concept map for this patient might look like this:

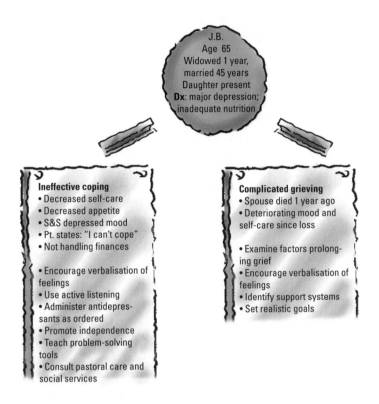

J.B.
Age 65
Widowed 1 year,
married 45 years
Daughter present
Dx: major depression;
inadequate nutrition

Ineffective coping
• Decreased self-care
• Decreased appetite
• S&S depressed mood
• Pt. states: "I can't cope"
• Not handling finances

• Encourage verbalisation of feelings
• Use active listening
• Administer antidepressants as ordered
• Promote independence
• Teach problem-solving tools
• Consult pastoral care and social services

Complicated grieving
• Spouse died 1 year ago
• Deteriorating mood and self-care since loss

• Examine factors prolonging grief
• Encourage verbalisation of feelings
• Identify support systems
• Set realistic goals

See *Sample mental health care plan*, pages 134 and 135 to see what the care plan might look like.

Sample mental health care plan

Here's an example of what the care plan might look like for the patient described in the text.

Nursing diagnosis 1

Ineffective coping related to sudden death of spouse 1 year ago as evidenced by lack of self-care and verbalisation of inability to cope.

Outcome

The patient will verbalise feelings about the death of her husband and demonstrate new coping mechanisms by discharge.

Interventions	Rationale
1. Encourage the patient to talk about her feelings.	1. Verbalising feelings makes the patient and others aware of what the patient is going through.
2. Use active listening and a calm, unhurried manner.	2. This approach conveys to the patient your concern and willingness to listen.
3. Administer antidepressants as ordered.	3. Medications may be essential to assist the patient with the mood disorder.
4. Encourage the patient to independently perform at least one activity of daily living each day.	4. Self-care helps improve patient outlook, self-worth, and independence.
5. Teach the patient problem-solving tools, such as the step-by step approach and weighing advantages and disadvantages.	5. Knowledge of problem-solving tools assists with day-to-day activities on discharge.
6. Allow the patient time to solve at least one simple problem per day on her own (such as what to eat or wear).	6. Successful problem-solving promotes independence and self-confidence.
7. Assist the patient in identifying problems or issues that she can't control or change.	7. Helping the patient realise her limitations decrease stress and feelings of incompetence.
8. Ensure patient is referred to Chaplaincy or counselling services as appropriate.	8. Spiritual guidance or assistance with other issues may be helpful as the patient identifies issues of concern.

(continued)

Sample mental health care plan (continued)

Nursing diagnosis 2

Complicated grieving related to loss of spouse as evidenced by depression, social isolation, inability to cope with activities of daily living (ADLs).

Outcome

The patient will verbalise feelings of grief and demonstrate use of new coping methods for managing her feelings by discharge.

Interventions	Rationale
1. Assess for factors that are prolonging the grieving process.	1. Identifying a problem will help to solve it.
2. Encourage the patient to talk about feelings of grief, anger and depression in individual and group therapy sessions.	2. Acknowledging feelings is first step to finding ways to deal with them.
3. Assist the patient in identifying her support systems.	3. Support systems can help patient in time of emotional need.
4. Discuss with the patient methods to cope with stresses such as focusing on living life 'one day at a time'.	4. Planning too far ahead can increase stress as new coping skills are developed.
5. Assist the patient in setting realistic goals.	5. Accomplishing short-term goals will help her gain a sense of control of her life.

Boy, oh boy!

A 10-year-old boy with cystic fibrosis, Bobby Young, is admitted to the hospital with upper respiratory infection and fever. His temperature is 38.5°C. He's coughing up copious amounts of yellowish green sputum. He's talkative but tires easily. His mother says his symptoms started about 2 days ago; she noticed that he'd gone to bed earlier because he was tired and that he appeared to be coughing more in the evening. She gave him an extra breathing treatment last night, but it didn't seem to help. The patient has been drinking his fluids well and taking his medications without any problems. His lung sounds on admission reveal rhonchi throughout the lower lobes. He has no acute shortness of breath and no other problems. His chest x-ray reveals no significant findings.

The concept map for this patient might look like this:

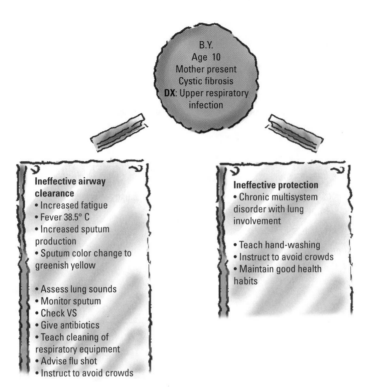

B.Y.
Age 10
Mother present
Cystic fibrosis
DX: Upper respiratory
infection

Ineffective airway clearance
• Increased fatigue
• Fever 38.5° C
• Increased sputum production
• Sputum color change to greenish yellow

• Assess lung sounds
• Monitor sputum
• Check VS
• Give antibiotics
• Teach cleaning of respiratory equipment
• Advise flu shot
• Instruct to avoid crowds

Ineffective protection
• Chronic multisystem disorder with lung involvement

• Teach hand-washing
• Instruct to avoid crowds
• Maintain good health habits

See *Sample children's care plan* to see what the care plan might look like. Note that this care plan addresses the patient's present infection and ongoing infection risk.

And many more ...

Throughout your nursing career, you're likely to create or encounter plenty of nursing care plans. Using the previous examples, and everything you've learned about care planning in this book, see if you can create your own care plan for the medical–surgical patient described in the *On the case.*

Sample children's care plan

Here's an example of what the care plan might look like for the patient described in the text.

Nursing diagnosis 1

Ineffective airway clearance related to acute respiratory infection as evidenced by increased amount of sputum, yellow-green sputum colour, increased fatigue and fever.

Outcome

The patient will demonstrate clear lung sounds, lack of fever and return to baseline energy level by discharge.

Interventions	Rationale
1. Assess lung sounds and respiratory pattern every shift and as needed.	1. Early recognition of worsening condition leads to early treatment and improved patient outcomes.
2. Assess amount, colour and consistency of sputum every shift.	2. Increased amounts, thickening and continued colour change of sputum can indicate worsening infection.
3. Assess vital signs every shift. Report deteriorating findings to the practitioner.	3. Increasing temperature and respirations indicate poor response to treatment.
4. Administer antibiotics as ordered.	4. Antibiotics help to fight infection.
5. Teach the patient and family proper cleaning of respiratory equipment.	5. Proper cleaning of respiratory equipment helps to prevent bacterial growth.
6. Teach the patient the importance of avoiding crowds during flu season and getting a flu vaccination.	6. Cystic fibrosis puts the patient at higher risk for infection. Avoiding crowds limits exposure to the flu. Getting a flu shot provides additional protection.

Nursing diagnosis 2

Ineffective protection related to cystic fibrosis as evidenced by ongoing sputum production, enzymatic disorder and increased risk of infection.

Outcome

The patient and family will verbalise understanding of instructions on risk reduction by discharge.

Interventions	Rationale
1. Reinforce with the patient and family that proactive hand-washing is a major defence against secondary infection.	1. Hand-washing prevents incidental exposure to infection.
2. Teach the patient and family to actively avoid crowded environments during flu season and to avoid people who are ill.	2. Active attention to environmental risks can decrease exposure to infectious agents.
3. Teach the patient to maintain healthy rest, nutrition and lung maintenance programs.	3. Healthy daily habits promote increased resistance to infectious agents.

On the case

Case study background

A 56-year-old male is admitted to the medical–surgical unit with chronic obstructive pulmonary disease (COPD) and pneumonia. He has shortness of breath and audible wheezes. He's unable to answer all of the medical history questions, so his wife answers for him while he sits, leaning over the bedside table. She says he has been coughing up more sputum the past 3 days and that it's green in colour. His vital signs are: oral temperature 38.5°C, pulse 115 beats/minute, respirations 28 breaths/minute and laboured with accessory muscle use, SaO_2 88% and blood pressure 142/68 mmHg. During the physical examination, the nurse notes oedema of both feet and an irregular heartbeat.

In accident and emergency (A&E) the patient was placed on 24% oxygen by face mask, I.V. sodium chloride 0.9% at 50 ml/hour, methylprednisolone sodium succinate (Solu-Medrone) 40 mg I.V. every six hours, erythromycin 500 mg I.V. four times a day, bed rest and nil-by-mouth status.

Critical thinking exercise

Complete a three-diagnosis care plan, including at least three interventions and rationales for each diagnosis, for this medical–surgical patient.

Nursing diagnosis 1

_____

Outcome

_____

Interventions	Rationale
1. _____	1. _____
2. _____	2. _____
3. _____	3. _____

Nursing diagnosis 2

_____

Outcome

_____

Interventions	Rationale
1. _____	1. _____
2. _____	2. _____
3. _____	3. _____

Nursing diagnosis 3

_____

Outcome

_____

Interventions	Rationale
1. _____	1. _____
2. _____	2. _____
3. _____	3. _____

Answer key

Five potential nursing diagnoses for this patient are given in the care plan on pages 143 to 145. See how many of your diagnoses, outcomes and interventions match. Did you think of a different diagnosis? You could be right! As long as your care plan was consistent with what you know about COPD and pneumonia, met the patient's profile and was logically thought out, you've probably developed a good care plan.

Nursing diagnosis 1

Impaired gas exchange related to inadequate ventilation and excessive mucus production.

Outcome

The patient will maintain adequate gas exchange as evidenced by return of arterial blood gas (ABG) values back to his baseline within 48 hours.

Interventions	Rationale
1. Assess and document respiratory rate and pattern, pulse oximetry every shift and ABGs as ordered. Report changes.	1. Early recognition of deteriorating respiratory function can improve patient outcomes.
2. Maintain low-flow oxygen therapy as ordered.	2. Oxygen therapy helps to correct hypoxemia. High oxygen saturation levels may diminish a COPD patient's respiratory drive and cause further retention of carbon dioxide.
3. Administer bronchodilators as ordered. Watch for adverse effects of tachycardia and arrhythmias.	3. Bronchodilators relax bronchial smooth muscle, improving air flow.
4. Assist the patient to orthopnaeic position as needed.	4. Orthopnaeic position promotes fuller lung expansion.

Nursing diagnosis 2

Ineffective airway clearance related to increased sputum production.

Outcome

The patient will have a patent airway as evidenced by decreased amounts of mucus by discharge.

Interventions	Rationale
1. Assess lung sounds and respiratory rate and pattern every 4 hours and as needed.	1. Rhonchi decrease the airflow patency of large airways. Increased respiratory rate and laboured breathing are signs of respiratory distress due to mucus plug or inadequate airway clearance.
2. Teach the patient effective coughing techniques.	2. Proper coughing techniques loosen mucus and ease expectoration, helping to conserve patient energy.
3. Teach the patient about adequate hydration (drinking at least 2500 ml of fluid per day, unless contraindicated).	3. Adequate hydration helps to thin secretions.
4. Encourage patient to carry out exercises prescribed by physiotherapists.	4. Chest physiotherapy helps to loosen secretions.
5. Monitor the patient's performance of incentive spirometry as ordered.	5. Incentive spirometry helps promote lung expansion.
6. Suction the patient to remove mucus from the back of the throat and mouth.	6. Thick secretions are difficult to cough out and the patient may not have the energy to do so.

Nursing diagnosis 3

Activity intolerance related to dyspnoea and inadequate oxygenation.

Outcome

The patient will perform activities of daily living (ADLs) with minimal assistance by discharge.

Interventions	Rationale
1. Monitor the severity of dyspnoea and oxygen saturation during patient activity.	1. Activity increases oxygen demand. Assessing these variables reveals the patient's tolerance of ADLs.
2. Stop or change any activity that causes worsening dyspnoea with increased heart rate.	2. Worsening dyspnoea with increased heart rate signals activity intolerance, which increases the patient's oxygen demand.
3. Maintain oxygen therapy with activity as needed.	3. Oxygen helps alleviate hypoxemia and helps to improve activity tolerance.
4. Schedule activities after breathing treatments.	4. Breathing treatments maximize lung function and improve activity tolerance.
5. Help the patient to gradually increase activities every day.	5. A gradual, steady increase in activity helps to improve respiratory and cardiac condition.
6. Teach the patient to avoid factors that increase oxygen demand, such as smoking, temperature extremes, excess weight and stress.	6. An increase in oxygen demand increases cardiac workload.
7. Teach the patient energy conservation techniques.	7. These techniques allow the patient to accomplish more with the limited energy he has.
8. Teach the patient pursed-lip and diaphragmatic breathing techniques and explain that he should use these techniques during activities.	8. These breathing techniques maximise lung function.

Nursing diagnosis 4

Risk of infection related to ineffective clearance of secretions.

Outcome

The patient will verbalise methods to reduce risk of infection by discharge.

Interventions	Rationale
1. Teach the patient proper hand-washing technique.	1. Good hand-washing is the single most important defence against the spread of infection.
2. Teach the patient how to care for and clean respiratory equipment at home.	2. Standing water in respiratory equipment can be a source of bacterial growth.
3. Teach the patient and family early signs of infection (increased sputum, change in sputum colour and increased dyspnoea).	3. Early detection leads to early treatment and decreases the risk of complications.
4. Teach the patient about the importance of getting a yearly flu vaccine.	4. The flu vaccine provides some immunity from infection.

Nursing diagnosis 5

Anxiety related to shortness of breath.

Outcome

The patient will verbalise decreased feelings of anxiety within 48 hours of admission.

Interventions	Rationale
1. Stay with the patient during episodes of shortness of breath and provide reassurance.	1. Having someone present during these episodes decreases patient anxiety.
2. Encourage the use of breathing techniques during episodes of shortness of breath and anxiety.	2. Successful use of breathing techniques helps to reduce anxiety.
3. Maintain a calm environment.	3. A calm environment promotes relaxation.
4. Teach the patient relaxation techniques, such as guided imagery and visualisation.	4. Relaxation techniques help to reduce anxiety.

Part II

Nursing diagnoses by medical diagnosis

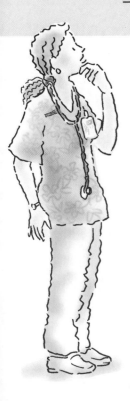

Just the facts

In this chapter, you'll learn:

♦ nursing diagnoses that correlate with common adult medical diagnoses in both acute and continuing care settings.

A look at medical–surgical diagnoses

This chapter covers medical and surgical problems that are common in adult patients. Each entry provides a list of a few of the major nursing diagnoses and related factors to be considered after your assessment of a patient with the particular medical diagnosis. Remember that the nursing diagnoses listed here represent some of the more specific needs most commonly associated with the medical condition; your patient may have different needs. For a majority of these diagnoses, the patient may also have a reduced inability to manage activities of daily living, in addition to the specific diagnoses listed in this section. You will also see that even where diagnoses and problems or needs are similar, there are still potentially many different ways of expressing this on a care plan. Remember, the important thing is to always consider and adhere to the principles of care planning and the nursing process.

> Remember that your nursing diagnoses should be specific to the patient—not necessarily the disorder.

Abdominal aortic aneurysm repair

- Acute pain related to surgical tissue trauma
- Anxiety related to threat to health status
- Decreased cardiac output related to:
  - changes in intravascular volume
  - increased systemic vascular resistance
  - third-space fluid shift

- Lack of knowledge about preoperative and postoperative care related to newly identified need for aortic surgery
- Ineffective breathing pattern related to:
  - effects of general anaesthesia
  - endotracheal intubation
  - presence of an abdominal incision

Abdominal injury

- Acute pain related to tissue trauma
- Deficient fluid volume related to active blood loss
- Fear related to unknown diagnosis and prognosis
- Risk of infection related to:
  - penetrating wound
  - potential bowel rupture

Acquired immunodeficiency syndrome (AIDS)

- Deficient fluid volume related to persistent diarrhoea associated with opportunistic infections
- Lack of knowledge about symptoms of disease progression, risk factors, transmission of disease, home care and treatment options related to lack of exposure to information
- Grieving related to uncertain prognosis and change in health status
- Inadequate nutritional intake related to:
  - anorexia
  - diarrhoea
  - medication adverse effects
  - nausea and vomiting
- Impaired gas exchange related to:
  - respiratory failure
  - ventilation–perfusion imbalance
- Impaired oral mucous membrane related to:
  - masses
  - opportunistic infections
- Impaired physical mobility related to:
  - fatigue and weakness
  - hypoxaemia
  - medication adverse effects
- Ineffective airway clearance related to pneumonia
- Ineffective breathing pattern related to fatigue
- Ineffective therapeutic regime management related to complexity of therapeutic regime
- Risk of compromised human dignity related to societal prejudice
- Risk of impaired skin integrity related to:
  - effects of immobility
  - medication reactions
  - opportunistic disease effects
  - poor nutritional status

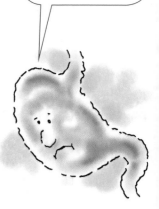

Abdominal injuries may be associated with pain or infection. Look for signs of these related problems in your patient.

- Risk of infection related to immunosuppression
- Altered sexual function related to:
  - depression
  - fatigue
  - fear of disease transmission
  - fear of rejection
- Social isolation related to:
  - associated societal stigma
  - contacts' fear of being infected
  - fear of infection from social contacts

Acute alcohol withdrawal

- Altered sensory perception (visual, auditory or tactile) related to underlying pathophysiological changes in the nervous system
- Altered thought processes related to disruption in cognitive operations
- Inadequate nutritional intake related to lack of food intake
- Risk of injury related to abrupt withdrawal of alcohol

Acute respiratory distress syndrome

- Deficient fluid volume related to active fluid volume loss
- Inadequate nutritional intake related to inability to ingest food due to mechanical ventilation
- Impaired gas exchange related to alveolar capillary membrane changes
- Impaired skin integrity related to immobility and decreased nutritional intake
- Impaired spontaneous ventilation related to respiratory muscle fatigue
- Impaired verbal communication related to physical barriers of mechanical ventilation
- Ineffective airway clearance related to retained secretions

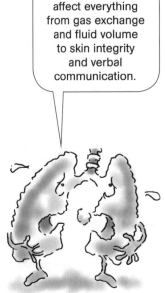

ARDS can affect everything from gas exchange and fluid volume to skin integrity and verbal communication.

Acute respiratory failure

- Activity intolerance related to respiratory distress and fatigue
- Anxiety related to sensation of severe shortness of breath
- Inability to independently maintain activities of daily living related to:
  - fatigue with exertion
  - shortness of breath at rest
- Inadequate nutritional intake related to shortness of breath
- Impaired gas exchange related to ventilation–perfusion imbalance
- Ineffective tissue perfusion (cardiopulmonary) related to impaired transport of oxygen across alveolar and capillary membranes

Adrenal hypofunction

- Decreased cardiac output related to altered heart rate
- Deficient fluid volume related to nausea, vomiting and diarrhoea
- Fatigue related to disease process

Alzheimer's disease

- Inability to independently maintain activities of daily living related to cognitive impairment
- Caregiver role strain related to the complexity and amount of care-giving tasks
- Chronic confusion related to degenerative loss of cerebral tissue
- Constipation related to:
  - inadequate diet
  - inadequate fluid intake
  - memory loss about toileting behaviour
- Inadequate nutritional intake related to:
  - difficulty swallowing
  - inadequate food intake
  - memory loss
- Impaired memory related to degenerative loss of cerebral tissue
- Risk of injury related to:
  - agnosia
  - aphasia
  - wandering behaviour
- Wandering related to cognitive impairment

Amputation

- Acute pain related to postoperative tissue, nerve and bone trauma
- Altered body image related to loss of a body part
- Impaired physical mobility related to loss of a body part
- Impaired skin integrity related to traumatic or surgical tissue removal
- Risk of injury related to altered mobility

Anaphylaxis

- Fear of dying related to acute respiratory distress
- Decreased cardiac output related to altered heart rate and hypotension
- Impaired gas exchange related to oedema of upper respiratory tract
- Ineffective tissue perfusion (cardiopulmonary, cerebral) related to impaired transport of oxygen across alveolar and capillary membranes

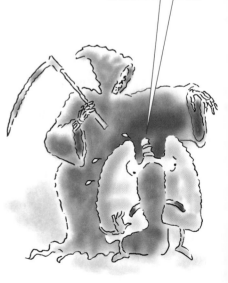

Oh no! Anaphylaxis can lead to respiratory-related death.

Anaemia

- Activity intolerance related to weakness, fatigue and shortness of breath
- Fatigue related to disease process
- Anxiety related to chronic fatigue and activity intolerance

- Inadequate nutritional intake related to:
  - anorexia
  - fatigue
  - lack of knowledge of need for specific nutrients (foliate, iron, vitamin B_{12})
- Ineffective protection related to decreased oxygen-carrying capacity of blood
- Risk of impaired skin integrity related to:
  - decreased mobility and bed rest
  - tissue hypoxia

Aneurysm, cerebral

- Acute pain related to aneurysm
- Compromised family coping related to unknown prognosis
- Decreased intracranial adaptive capacity related to increased intracranial pressure from brain haemorrhage
- Risk of acute confusion related to moderate bleeding of cerebral artery into the brain

Aneurysm, femoral and popliteal

- Acute pain related to:
  - compression of nerves
  - oedema
  - ischaemia
- Lack of knowledge about preoperative and postoperative care related to lack of exposure to information
- Ineffective tissue perfusion (peripheral) related to thrombus formation and ischemia

Aneurysm, thoracic aortic

- Acute pain related to thoracic aortic aneurysm
- Ineffective tissue perfusion (cardiopulmonary) related to aortic insufficiency
- Risk of deficient fluid volume related to compromised regulatory mechanisms

Aneurysm, ventricular

- Fear of dying related to risk of life-threatening rupture
- Decreased cardiac output related to arrhythmias
- Ineffective tissue perfusion (cardiopulmonary) related to heart failure

Angina pectoris

- Activity intolerance related to development of chest pain on exertion
- Anxiety related to shortness of breath
- Decreased cardiac output related to reduced stroke volume

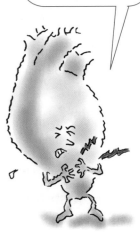

Angina pectoris can lead some patients to be intolerant of exercise.

- Lack of knowledge about cardiac diagnostic procedures related to new onset of angina
- Ineffective management and reduction of risk factors related to lack of knowledge about condition

Ankylosing spondylitis

- Activity intolerance related to pain and inflammation of joints
- Chronic pain related to deteriorating bone and cartilage of joints
- Inability to engage in normal activities of daily living related to pain, stiffness and limitation of spinal motion
- Disturbed sensory perception (visual) related to eye inflammation

Appendicitis

- Acute pain related to inflammatory process
- Nausea related to peritoneal inflammation
- Risk of infection related to:
  - possible rupture of appendix
  - surgical incision

Arterial occlusive disease

- Acute pain related to arterial occlusion
- Lack of knowledge about disease and treatment options related to lack of exposure to information
- Altered sensory perception (tactile) related to arterial occlusion
- Ineffective tissue perfusion (peripheral) related to reduced arterial blood flow

Atelectasis

- Anxiety related to shortness of breath
- Impaired gas exchange related to alveolar-capillary membrane changes
- Ineffective airway clearance related to excessive mucus

Basal cell epithelioma

- Altered body image related to cancerous lesion
- Lack of knowledge about reduction of risk factors related to new diagnosis

Bell's palsy

- Altered body image related to unilateral facial weakness
- Altered sensory perception related to altered sensory reception
- Social isolation related to altered body image

Benign prostatic hyperplasia

- Impaired urinary elimination related to obstruction by enlarged prostate
- Risk of deficient fluid volume related to postoperative bleeding

- Altered sexual function related to postsurgical recovery time, retrograde ejaculation and anxiety
- Urinary retention related to physiological changes

Bladder cancer

- Lack of knowledge about disease and treatment options related to lack of exposure to information
- Fear related to unknown prognosis
- Impaired tissue integrity related to radiation or chemotherapy
- Impaired urinary elimination related to bladder irritability and pain
- Low self-esteem (postoperative) related to self-consciousness and disturbed self-image after urinary diversion surgery

Blepharitis

- Altered body image related to inflammation of margins of eyelids
- Effective therapeutic regime management related to ability to manage symptoms
- Impaired skin integrity related to inflammation

Bone tumour

- Acute pain related to pressure from tumour growth
- Anxiety related to change in health status
- Impaired physical mobility related to tumour growth or postoperative healing response
- Impaired skin integrity related to surgical incision for tumour removal

Botulism

- Fear of dying related to life-threatening disorder
- Deficient fluid volume related to vomiting and diarrhoea
- Ineffective breathing pattern related to respiratory muscle failure

Brain abscess

- Acute pain related to oedema and necrosis
- Ineffective tissue perfusion (cerebral) related to oedema and necrosis
- Risk of acute confusion related to neurological impairment
- Risk of injury related to neurological impairment

Brain tumour

- Anxiety related to:
  - deterioration of physical and mental function
  - risks of treatment options
- Decreased intracranial adaptive capacity related to brain tissue injury

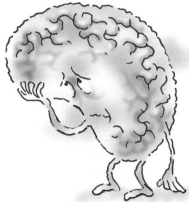

Did someone say brain tumour? Now I'm getting anxious!

- Altered thought processes related to brain mass injury
- Impaired verbal communication related to damage to speech centre
- Risk of acute confusion related to tissue damage from brain mass
- Risk of injury related to increased seizure potential and neuromuscular effects of brain tissue damage

Breast cancer

- Inadequate knowledge about treatment choices related to lack of information giving
- Altered body image related to breast surgery
- Fatigue related to effects of disease and treatments
- Impaired skin integrity related to incision following breast surgery
- Altered sexual patterns related to perceived loss of attractiveness after mastectomy
- Stress overload related to family needs while physically and emotionally taxed

Bronchiectasis

- Inadequate nutritional intake related to inadequate food intake due to illness
- Ineffective breathing pattern related to chronic abnormal dilation of bronchi and destruction of bronchial walls
- Risk of infection related to repeated damage to bronchial walls

Buerger's disease

- Lack of knowledge about risk factors and treatment options related to new diagnosis
- Altered body image related to disease
- Ineffective tissue perfusion (peripheral) related to decreased blood flow to the feet and legs
- Lack of education about smoking cessation related to new diagnosis

Burns

- Acute pain related to tissue destruction and exposure of nerves in partially destroyed tissue
- Compromised family coping related to prolonged disease or disability
- Contamination related to infective agents at place of injury
- Altered body image related to potential scarring
- Inadequate nutritional intake related to increased metabolic needs of burn healing
- Impaired gas exchange related to airway burns and carbon monoxide inhalation
- Impaired physical mobility related to movement limitations from scar tissue or burn treatments

- Powerlessness related to illness
- Risk of deficient fluid volume related to active loss through disrupted skin
- Risk of imbalanced body temperature related to infection
- Risk of impaired skin integrity related to nonadherence of graft and impaired donor site healing
- Risk of infection related to:
  - decreased perfusion
  - exposure to contamination
  - impaired immune response
  - loss of protective integument
- Risk of injury related to continued exposure to heat or chemicals

Cancer

- Activity intolerance related to weakness from:
  - altered protein metabolism
  - cachexia
  - hypoxia
  - muscle wasting
- Anxiety related to diagnosis, treatment effects and prognosis
- Chronic pain related to:
  - chemotherapy side effects
  - metastasis
  - primary disease
- Inadequate nutritional intake related to:
  - anorexia
  - changes in taste sensation
  - stomatitis
- Impaired urinary elimination related to haemorrhagic cystitis from chemotherapy
- Altered sexuality related to alterations in body image
- Risk of constipation related to opioid use
- Risk of infection related to immunosuppression from chemotherapy and malnutrition
- Risk of peripheral neurovascular dysfunction related to peripheral neuropathies caused by chemotherapy
- Risk of low self-esteem related to:
  - hair loss
  - role changes
  - weight loss
- Sleep deprivation related to:
  - alterations in patterns of elimination
  - anxiety
  - fear of dying while sleeping
  - other sequelae of cancer
  - pain

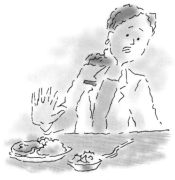

Patients with cancer can experience imbalanced nutrition as a result of anorexia, changes in taste and anxiety. Nothing for me right now, thanks.

Candidiasis

- Impaired oral mucous membrane related to fungal infection in mouth
- Impaired skin integrity related to fungal infection
- Ineffective thermoregulation related to systemic infection
- Risk of impaired liver function related to fluconazole (Diflucan) or other specific systemic antifungal agents

Cardiac arrhythmias

- Activity intolerance related to shortness of breath or chest pain
- Anxiety related to change in health status
- Decreased cardiac output related to altered contractility of heart muscle
- Lack of knowledge about disease and treatment options related to lack of exposure to information
- Fatigue related to arrhythmias
- Fear related to decreased confidence in health status
- Ineffective coping related to inadequate level of control over illness recurrence
- Ineffective tissue perfusion (cardiopulmonary) related to impaired cardiac cycle and blood oxygenation

Cardiac surgery

- Acute confusion related to:
  - anaesthesia
  - cerebral ischaemia or infarction
  - sensory overload from intensive care unit environment
- Deficient fluid volume related to blood loss
- Lack of knowledge about postoperative care requirements related to complex therapeutic regime
- Dysfunctional ventilatory weaning response related to respiratory complications postoperatively
- Impaired gas exchange related to:
  - alveolar collapse
  - increased pulmonary shunt
  - increased secretions
  - pain

Cardiac tamponade

- Decreased cardiac output related to altered preload
- Fear of dying related to life-threatening disorder
- Ineffective breathing pattern related to cardiac tamponade

Cardiogenic shock

- Activity intolerance related to:
  - diminished cardiovascular reserve

- hypoxaemia
- weakness
- Decreased cardiac output related to heart rate abnormalities or diminished contractility
- Excess fluid volume related to compromised regulatory mechanisms
- Impaired gas exchange related to ventilation–perfusion imbalance

Cardiomyopathy

- Anxiety related to deterioration in health status (medication effects and adverse effects)
- Decreased cardiac output related to arrhythmias and ineffective pump function
- Lack of knowledge about disease and treatment related to change in health status
- Ineffective breathing pattern related to disease process

Carotid endarterectomy

- Anxiety related to threat to health status
- Lack of knowledge about procedure related to unfamiliarity with hospital protocol
- Impaired gas exchange related to airway obstruction from tracheal compression or aspiration
- Risk of infection related to surgical incision

Carpal tunnel syndrome

- Acute pain related to nerve compression
- Bathing or hygiene self-care deficit related to pain
- Risk of peripheral neurovascular dysfunction related to disease process

Cataract

- Inadequate knowledge about disease and treatment option related to lack of exposure to information
- Altered sensory perception (visual) related to cataract
- Impaired physical mobility related to fear of injury
- Risk of injury related to impaired vision

Cerebral contusion

- Acute pain related to headache after trauma
- Altered sensory perception (auditory, olfactory, visual) related to bruising of brain tissue
- Risk of acute confusion related to brain injury
- Risk of accidental injury related to confusion

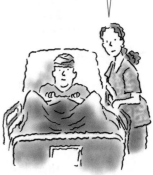

Disturbances in auditory, olfactory and visual perception can result from cerebral contusion.

Cervical cancer

- Acute pain related to tumour invasion
- Inadequate knowledge about disease and treatment options related to lack of exposure to information
- Altered body image related to weight loss
- Fatigue related to cancer process and treatment effects
- Altered sexual function related to postcoital pain and bleeding

Chest injury, blunt

- Acute pain related to injury
- Anxiety related to impaired oxygenation
- Impaired spontaneous ventilation related to blunt trauma
- Ineffective breathing pattern related to chest wall injury

Chlamydia

- Lack of knowledge about disease and treatment options related to need for health promotion
- Altered patterns of sexual activity related to fear of spreading infection
- Lack of education about safe sexual practices related to prevention of reoccurrence
- Risk of infection related to untreated partners

Cholecystectomy

- Acute pain related to gallbladder inflammation
- Inadequate nutritional intake related to:
  - altered lipid metabolism
  - increased nutritional needs during healing
  - nasogastric (NG) suction
  - postoperative nil-by-mouth (NBM) status
  - preoperative nausea and vomiting
- Impaired oral mucous membrane related to NBM status and possible NG suction
- Ineffective breathing pattern related to pain from high abdominal incision
- Risk of infection (postoperative) related to obstruction of external biliary drainage tube

Cholecystitis

- Acute pain related to gallbladder inflammation or presence of stones
- Inadequate nutritional intake related to attacks following meals
- Risk of infection related to complications of disease

Chronic alcoholism

- Altered family relationships related to alcohol abuse
- Inadequate nutritional intake related to lack of food intake

- Ineffective coping related to:
  - anger
  - denial
  - dependence
- Ineffective therapeutic regime management related to denial of problem
- Risk of impaired liver function related to alcohol intake
- Risk of violence and aggression related to:
  - disorientation
  - impaired judgement
- Risk-prone health behaviour related to alcohol abuse

Chronic obstructive pulmonary disease

- Activity intolerance related to shortness of breath
- Adult failure to thrive related to fatigue and chronic dyspnoea of severe disease
- Lack of knowledge about disease processes and treatment related to complexity of disorder
- Inadequate nutritional intake related to shortness of breath during and after meals
- Impaired gas exchange related to impaired excretion of carbon dioxide
- Impaired coping at home related to inadequate support systems and inability to do tasks due to disease process
- Ineffective breathing pattern related to fatigue, or blunting of respiratory drive
- Altered patterns of sexual activity related to:
  - adverse reactions to medications
  - change in body image
  - change in relationship with spouse or partner
  - deconditioning
  - shortness of breath
- Insomnia related to:
  - anxiety
  - bronchodilator's stimulant effect
  - depression
  - shortness of breath

Cirrhosis

- Altered family relationships related to alcohol addiction
- Excess fluid volume related to fluid retention
- Inadequate nutritional intake related to:
  - gastrointestinal (GI) symptoms (anorexia, nausea, vomiting, diarrhoea)
  - inability to absorb nutrients
- Impaired gas exchange related to ventilation–perfusion imbalance
- Risk of acute confusion related to increasing ammonia levels
- Risk of impaired liver function related to alcohol addiction
- Risk of impaired skin integrity related to oedema and pruritus

Clostridium difficile infection

- Anxiety related to change in health status
- Risk of deficient fluid volume related to diarrhoea
- Risk of impaired skin integrity related to diarrhoea
- Risk of infection related to inadequate defences

Colorectal cancer

- Constipation related to GI obstruction
- Diarrhoea related to inflammation or malabsorption
- Fatigue related to malnutrition or anaemia
- Inadequate nutritional intake related to inability to absorb nutrients
- Risk of deficient fluid volume related to diarrhoea or bleeding
- Risk of spiritual distress related to potential life-threatening diagnosis

Colostomy

- Lack of knowledge about care of the stoma related to unfamiliarity
- Altered body image related to loss of control over faecal elimination
- Risk of impaired skin integrity related to faecal contamination of skin
- Altered sexual function related to change in body image

Concussion

- Disturbed sensory perception (visual) related to a blow to the head
- Nausea related to blow to the head
- Risk of injury related to dizziness and lethargy

Conjunctivitis

- Risk of impaired skin integrity related to eye discharge and tearing
- Risk of infection related to contagious disease and ability to spread to other eye or other people
- Risk of low self-esteem related to hyperemia of eyes

Cor pulmonale

- Activity intolerance related to exertional dyspnoea
- Decreased cardiac output related to decreased stroke volume
- Grieving related to poor prognosis
- Impaired gas exchange related to pulmonary capillary destruction

Corneal abrasion

- Acute pain related to eye injury
- Altered sensory perception (visual) related to eye injury
- Risk of injury related to poor visual acuity

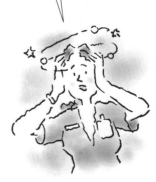

A patient with a concussion is at risk of injuries related to dizziness and lethargy. Now that's a blow to the head!

Corneal ulcer

- Altered sensory perception (visual) related to corneal ulcer
- Risk of infection related to inadequate primary defences
- Risk of injury related to visual blurring

Coronary artery disease

- Anxiety related to angina
- Decreased cardiac output related to diminished coronary blood flow
- Lack of education about lifestyle changes related to perceived ability to decrease risk factors
- Ineffective tissue perfusion (cardiopulmonary) related to atherosclerosis

Craniotomy

- Lack of knowledge about impending craniotomy related to lack of exposure to information
- Altered body image related to hair loss and possible disruption of motor function
- Risk of deficient fluid volume related to:
  - diuretic therapy
  - fluid restriction
  - GI suction
  - hyperthermia
- Risk of infection related to invasive techniques (surgery, continuous intracranial monitoring, ventricular drains)
- Risk of injury related to:
  - decreased level of consciousness
  - drug therapy
  - effect of anaesthetics
  - seizures

Crohn's disease

- Acute pain related to bowel inflammation
- Compromised family coping related to chronic disease
- Diarrhoea related to bowel inflammation
- Nausea related to bowel inflammation
- Risk of imbalanced fluid volume related to diarrhoea
- Risk of infection related to invasive procedures (surgery, home infusions)

Cushing's syndrome

- Disturbed body image related to secondary effects of excessive corticosteroid levels
- Excess fluid volume related to high serum corticosteroid levels

- Risk of impaired skin integrity related to secondary effects of medications
- Risk of infection related to the immunosuppressive action of glucocorticoids
- Risk of unstable glucose level related to the anti-insulin properties of glucocorticoids

Dermatitis

- Chronic low self-esteem related to poor body image
- Impaired skin integrity related to inflammation, itching or lesions of the skin
- Risk of infection related to inadequate primary defences

Diabetes (Types I and II)

- Compromised family coping related to chronic disease
- Lack of knowledge about diabetes related to complex chronic disease
- Ineffective management of therapeutic regime related to:
    - ineffective coping with chronic disorders
    - lack of material resources
    - lack of support
- Ineffective tissue perfusion (renal, peripheral) related to complications of disease
- Risk of inadequate nutritional intake related to need for diabetic diet
- Risk of unstable glucose level related to:
    - poor monitoring of blood glucose levels
    - nonconcordance with treatment and management regime

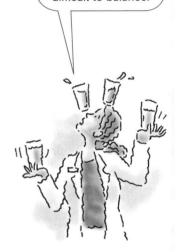

Watch for signs of dehydration in a patient with diabetes. Fluid volume can be difficult to balance.

Diabetic ketoacidosis

- Deficient fluid volume related to osmotic diuresis or vomiting
- Lack of knowledge about treatment related to lack of exposure to complex disease and therapy information
- Risk of injury related to:
    - acidosis
    - cerebral dehydration
    - decreased perfusion
    - hypoxemia
- Risk of unstable glucose level related to decreased cellular glucose uptake and use

Dislocation and subluxation

- Acute pain related to damage to tissue
- Anxiety related to pain and treatment
- Impaired physical mobility related to joint injury and pain

Disseminated intravascular coagulation

- Acute pain related to:
  - bleeding into organ or joint capsules
  - haematomas
  - tissue ischaemia
- Deficient fluid volume related to haemorrhage
- Fear related to unfamiliarity with hospital environment
- Impaired gas exchange related to hypoxaemia
- Impaired skin integrity related to capillary fragility

Diverticulitis

- Acute pain related to:
  - bowel infection or perforation
  - inflammation
- Constipation related to lack of roughage in diet
- Deficient fluid volume related to active loss and poor intake
- Diarrhoea related to inflammation and infection

Drug overdose

- Hopelessness related to:
  - overwhelming feelings of despair
  - inadequate coping strategies
  - low self-esteem
- Ineffective airway clearance related to:
  - decreased or absent gag reflex
  - lavage procedures
  - obstruction by tongue
  - reduced alertness
  - vomiting
- Risk-prone health behaviour related to fluctuations in emotional status

Duodenal ulcer

- Chronic pain related to:
  - excessive motility of upper GI tract
  - increased hydrochloric acid secretion
  - increased spasm
  - inflammation of the duodenum
  - intragastric pressure
- Inadequate nutritional intake related to:
  - dysphagia
  - mouth soreness
  - nausea and vomiting

- Risk of deficient fluid volume related to:
  - diarrhoea
  - GI haemorrhage
  - vomiting

Encephalitis

- Acute pain related to increased intracranial pressure
- Altered thought processes related to cerebral oedema
- Hyperthermia related to infection
- Impaired physical mobility related to possible coma

Endocarditis

- Activity intolerance related to fatigue and weakness
- Decreased cardiac output related to bacterial or fungal invasion of heart
- Hyperthermia related to infection

Endometriosis

- Acute pain related to inflammation and adhesions of endometrial tissue
- Lack of knowledge about disease and treatment options related to lack of exposure to information
- Altered sexual function related to pain

Epididymitis

- Acute pain related to infection
- Risk of infection related to inadequate primary defences
- Altered sexual function related to pain, swelling and tenderness of groin area

Epilepsy

- Lack of knowledge about disease related to lack of exposure to information
- Fatigue related to antiseizure medication side effect
- Lack of education about management of therapeutic regime related to chronic nature of the illness
- Risk of caregiver role strain related to worry and fear about diagnosis
- Risk of compromised human dignity related to seizures

Escherichia coli and other *Enterobacteriaceae* infections

- Acute pain related to crampy diarrhoea
- Deficient fluid volume related to loss through diarrhoea and vomiting
- Diarrhoea related to infection

Femoral popliteal bypass

- Acute pain related to surgical incision
- Impaired physical mobility related to surgery and pre-existing disability
- Impaired skin integrity related to surgical incision and pre-existing stasis ulcers
- Ineffective tissue perfusion (peripheral) related to arterial insufficiency
- Risk of infection related to inadequate primary defences (broken skin)

Fibromyalgia syndrome

- Chronic pain related to illness
- Fatigue related to musculoskeletal pain and sleep disturbance
- Insomnia related to pain

Gastric cancer

- Deficient fluid volume related to vomiting and decreased fluid intake
- Delayed surgical recovery related to decreased nutrition and primary defences
- Inadequate nutritional intake: Less than body requirements related to:
  – a feeling of fullness after eating
  – dyspepsia
  – epigastric discomfort
- Risk of spiritual distress related to cancer diagnosis and prognosis

Gastritis

- Acute pain related to inflammation
- Lack of knowledge about prevention and treatment related to lack of exposure to smoking, diet information and medication use
- Nausea related to gastric irritation
- Lack of education regarding appropriate diet related to long-term management of disease.

Gastroenteritis

- Acute pain related to intestinal flu
- Nausea related to bacteria, parasites and virus in intestine
- Risk of deficient fluid volume related to nausea and vomiting
- Risk of imbalanced body temperature related to infection

Gastroesophageal reflux

- Chronic pain related to reflux of gastric and duodenal contents into oesophagus
- Lack of knowledge about prevention and management related to lack of exposure to information
- Risk of aspiration related to reflux

GI haemorrhage

- Deficient fluid volume related to active bleeding
- Lack of knowledge about potential recurrent bleeding related to unfamiliarity with disorder
- Fear related to sight of blood and distressing physical symptoms
- Risk of injury related to:
  - accumulation of toxins
  - electrolyte imbalance
  - inadequate organ perfusion
  - ulcer perforation
  - undetected bleeding

Glaucoma

- Anxiety related to progression of disease
- Lack of knowledge about eye drop administration procedure related to lack of previous experience
- Disturbed sensory perception (visual) related to high intraocular pressure and damage to optic nerve
- Risk of injury related to loss of peripheral vision

Glomerulonephritis

- Excess fluid volume related to oliguria
- Inadequate nutritional intake related to disease processes
- Ineffective tissue perfusion (renal) related to disease process
- Risk of infection related to inadequate defences

Goiter

- Altered body image related to neck distension
- Impaired swallowing related to swelling and distension of neck
- Ineffective breathing pattern related to compression of trachea

Gonorrhoea

- Altered sexual patterns related to fear of spreading infection
- Risk of infection related to inadequate primary resources
- Risk of low self-esteem related to infection
- Lack of education about safe sexual practices related to the need to prevent reoccurrence

Gout

- Activity intolerance related to painful joints
- Acute pain related to urate deposits in joints
- Altered body image related to joint deformity

Granulocytopenia, lymphocytopenia

- Lack of knowledge about disease and treatment options related to lack of exposure to information
- Fatigue related to low white blood cell (WBC) count
- Hyperthermia related to infection
- Risk of infection related to low WBC count

Guillain–Barré syndrome

- Inability to independently maintain activities of daily living related to muscle weakness and paralysis
- Fear related to sudden onset of illness
- Impaired spontaneous ventilation related to muscle weakness and paralysis
- Ineffective airway clearance related to neuromuscular dysfunction
- Risk of urge urinary incontinence related to muscle weakness

Headache

- Acute pain related to vascular, muscle contraction
- Fatigue related to headache
- Ineffective coping related to recurrence of headaches

Hearing loss

- Altered sensory perception (auditory) related to hearing loss
- Lack of education about alternative communication strategies related to ongoing hearing loss
- Risk of injury related to not hearing danger signs in environment

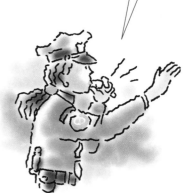

Your patient's hearing loss can affect his ability to hear danger signals in the environment, putting him at risk for injury.

Heart failure

- Decreased cardiac output related to:
  - altered heart rhythm
  - decreased contractility
  - fluid volume overload
  - increased after-load
- Lack of knowledge about treatment regime related to lack of exposure to information
- Excess fluid volume related to:
  - decreased myocardial contractility
  - decreased renal perfusion
  - increased sodium and water retention
- Inadequate nutritional intake related to decreased appetite and un-palatability of low-sodium diet
- Ineffective breathing pattern related to fatigue

- Ineffective therapeutic regime management related to:
  - complexity of regime
  - health beliefs
  - negative relationship with caregivers
- Powerlessness related to illness

Haemophilia

- Anxiety related to risk of acute bleeding
- Ineffective protection related to abnormal blood profile
- Risk of injury related to lack of awareness of environmental dangers
- Risk of trauma related to external factors

Haemorrhoids

- Acute pain related to inflammation of haemorrhoid veins
- Constipation related to pain
- Lack of knowledge about activities that increase pressure related to the need to prevent reoccurrence

Haemothorax

- Acute pain related to blood in pleural cavity
- Anxiety related to acute shortness of breath
- Fear related to sudden onset of injury
- Ineffective breathing pattern related to blood in pleural cavity

Hepatic encephalopathy

- Deficient fluid volume related to active loss
- Disturbed thought processes related to ammonia intoxication of the brain
- Risk of impaired liver function related to alcohol abuse

Hepatitis

- Acute pain related to inflammation of the liver
- Lack of knowledge about home care, disease process and prevention of recurrence related to lack of exposure to information
- Fatigue related to disease process
- Inadequate nutritional intake related to anorexia, diarrhoea, nausea or vomiting
- Nausea related to GI irritation
- Risk of activity intolerance related to increased fatigue
- Risk of deficient fluid volume related to vomiting and diarrhoea
- Risk of impaired skin integrity related to:
  - frequent diarrhoea
  - prolonged bed rest
  - pruritus

Herniated disc

- Activity intolerance related to pain
- Acute pain related to impingement on spinal nerve roots

Herpes simplex

- Acute pain related to cold sores and fever blisters
- Chronic low self-esteem related to skin lesions
- Altered patterns of sexual activity related to fear of spreading infection to sexual partner
- Sexual dysfunction related to sexually transmitted disease (herpes simplex 2)

Herpes zoster

- Acute pain related to inflammation of the dorsal root ganglia
- Chronic pain related to neuralgia
- Hyperthermia related to infection
- Impaired skin integrity related to localised vesicular skin lesions

Hiatus hernia

- Acute pain related to displacement or stretching of the stomach
- Inadequate knowledge about treatment options related to lack of exposure to information
- Impaired swallowing related to oesophagitis, ulcers or strictures

Hodgkin's disease

- Fatigue related to weight loss and disease process
- Grieving related to perceived potential for loss of life
- Hyperthermia related to immunosuppression
- Ineffective protection related to Hodgkin's disease

Huntington's disease

- Inability to independently maintain activities of daily living related to physical deterioration
- Bowel incontinence related to neuromuscular impairment
- Caregiver role strain related to complexity and amount of care giving activities
- Altered thought processes related to brain involvement
- Impaired physical mobility related to neuromuscular impairment
- Impaired verbal communication related to dysarthria

Hydronephrosis

- Acute pain related to physical obstruction of urine flow
- Impaired urinary elimination related to obstruction of urine flow
- Risk of infection related to obstruction of urine flow

Hyperaldosteronism

- Inadequate knowledge about disease related to lack of exposure to information
- Fatigue related to hypokalaemia
- Impaired urinary elimination related to polyuria and polydipsia
- Risk of unstable glucose level related to hypokalaemia

Hyperparathyroidism

- Acute pain related to hypocalcaemia, which causes bone tenderness, pancreatitis and peptic ulcers
- Hopelessness related to deteriorating condition
- Inadequate nutritional intake related to nausea and vomiting

Hypertension

- Decreased cardiac output related to decreased stroke volume
- Excess fluid volume related to compromised regulatory mechanisms
- Ineffective therapeutic regime management related to deficient knowledge
- Nonconcordance (treatment and management regime) related to health beliefs and cultural influences

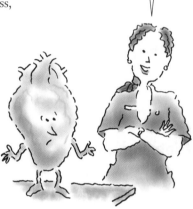

Patients with hypertension can nonconcordant as a result of health beliefs or cultural influences.

Hypoglycaemia

- Fatigue related to hypoglycaemia
- Ineffective management of therapeutic regime related to complexity of the disease and lack of knowledge
- Risk of injury related to:
  - excessive exercise
  - inappropriate exogenous insulin use
  - lack of food

Hypoparathyroidism

- Decreased cardiac output related to cardiac arrhythmias
- Inadequate nutritional intake related to inability to ingest foods due to dysphagia
- Ineffective coping related to situational crisis

Hypothyroidism

- Decreased cardiac output related to cardiac arrhythmias
- Altered body image related to periorbital oedema and upper eyelid droop
- Altered thought processes related to decreasing mental stability and forgetfulness
- Risk of imbalanced body temperature related to decreased sensitivity of thermo receptors

Hypovolaemic shock

- Decreased cardiac output related to altered heart rate and rhythm
- Impaired gas exchange related to ventilation–perfusion imbalance
- Ineffective coping related to threat to life
- Ineffective tissue perfusion (cerebral, cardiopulmonary, renal, peripheral) related to hypovolemia
- Risk of deficient fluid volume related to:
    - disease processes
    - iatrogenic interventions
    - surgical interventions
- Risk of injury related to complications from ischemia

Ileal conduit urinary diversion

- Lack of knowledge about the care of an ileal conduit related to lack of exposure to information
- Altered body image related to urinary diversion
- Impaired urinary elimination related to creation of an ileal conduit
- Risk of infection related to GI or genitourinary anastomosis breakdown or leakage
- Altered sexual function related to cystectomy and possible ejaculatory incompetence with prostatectomy

Incontinence

- Risk of impaired skin integrity due to contact between urine or faeces and the skin
- Altered body image related to incontinence
- Anxiety due to inability to manage elimination needs independently

Infertility

- Complicated grieving related to multiple miscarriages
- Ineffective coping related to uncertainty of future pregnancies
- Situational low self-esteem related to infertility

Inflammatory bowel disease

- Chronic pain related to abdominal distension
- Deficient fluid volume related to decreased fluid intake and increased fluid loss through diarrhoea
- Inadequate nutritional intake related to:
    - decreased nutrient intake
    - increased nutrient loss
    - possible decreased bowel absorption
- Impaired skin integrity related to frequent stools and altered nutritional status

- Altered sexual patterns related to diminished physical energy and persistence of uncomfortable physical symptoms
- Insomnia related to:
    - anxiety related to hospitalisation
    - nocturnal defecation
    - uncomfortable sensations
- Risk of infection related to:
    - bowel perforation
    - general debilitation
    - immunosuppression
- Social isolation related to dependent behaviour

Influenza

- Hyperthermia related to infection
- Risk of imbalanced fluid volume related to fever, cough, decreased oral intake
- Risk of infection related to inadequate primary and secondary defences to prevent secondary bacterial invasion

Inguinal hernia

- Acute pain related to tension on herniated contents
- Ineffective tissue perfusion (GI) related to diversion of bowel through hernia
- Risk of infection related to complete obstruction

Intestinal obstruction

- Acute pain related to abdominal distension
- Constipation related to intestinal obstruction
- Ineffective tissue perfusion (GI) related to obstruction
- Risk of deficient fluid volume related to intestinal obstruction

Joint replacement

- Acute pain related to surgery
- Impaired physical mobility related to joint surgery
- Risk of infection related to incision

Kaposi's sarcoma

- Acute pain related to lesions that break down or impinge on nerves and organs
- Grieving related to threat of death in advanced disease and when associated with human immunodeficiency virus
- Impaired skin integrity related to disease process
- Ineffective breathing pattern related to bronchial blockage and hypoventilation

Kidney transplant

- Acute pain related to frequent invasive procedures and surgery
- Altered body image related to effects of steroid therapy
- Excess fluid volume related to function of transplanted kidney
- Ineffective coping related to sensory overload
- Noncompliance (drug regime) related to adverse drug effects and complicated multiple drug regime
- Anxiety related to fear of organ rejection
- Risk of infection related to immunosuppression

Laminectomy

- Acute pain related to:
  - immobility
  - muscle spasm
  - paresthesia secondary to surgical trauma and postoperative oedema
- Lack of knowledge about preoperative and postoperative care related to lack of exposure to information
- Ineffective tissue perfusion (renal) related to:
  - anesthesia
  - anxiety
  - cord oedema
  - injury to the spinal nerve roots innervating the bladder
  - opioids
  - pain
  - supine positioning
- Risk of deficient fluid volume related to:
  - blood loss during surgery
  - haemorrhage at the incision site
  - retroperitoneal haemorrhage
  - vascular injury

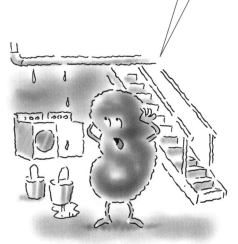

Your patient may have excess fluid volume related to the function of his transplanted kidney. My pail runneth over…

Laryngeal cancer

- Acute pain on swallowing related to pressure from tumour
- Anxiety related to potentially life limiting illness
- Inadequate nutritional intake related to impaired swallowing
- Impaired swallowing related to tumour
- Impaired verbal communication related to laryngectomy

Legionnaires' disease

- Diarrhoea related to infection
- Fatigue related to infection
- Hyperthermia related to infection

- Ineffective airway clearance related to increased mucus production
- Risk of infection related to inadequate immune defences to prevent secondary bacterial invasion

Leukaemia

- Activity intolerance related to:
  – depressed nutritional status
  – fatigue secondary to rapid destruction of leukaemia cells
  – tissue hypoxia secondary to anaemia
- Acute pain related to physical, biological or chemical agents
- Lack of knowledge about the choice of treatment options related to lack of exposure to information
- Fatigue related to rapid destruction of leukaemia cells
- Hopelessness related to prognosis
- Inadequate nutritional intake related to:
  – anorexia
  – chemotherapy
  – nausea
  – taste perception changes
  – vomiting
- Impaired oral mucous membrane related to:
  – cytotoxic effects of chemotherapy
  – immunosuppression secondary to disease
- Ineffective coping related to uncertain prognosis and multiple disease- and treatment-induced losses
- Ineffective protection related to severe immunosuppression associated with bone marrow transplantation or peripheral stem cell transplantation protocol
- Risk of deficient fluid volume related to potential haemorrhage
- Risk of infection related to immunosuppression

Liver abscess

- Acute pain related to liver abscess
- Anxiety related to change in health status
- Impaired gas exchange related to abnormal breathing rate and rhythm due to pain
- Risk of imbalanced body temperature related to infection

Liver failure

- Inadequate nutritional intake related to catabolism caused by liver disease
- Impaired skin integrity related to:
  – ascites
  – increased bleeding tendencies
  – jaundice
  – malnutrition

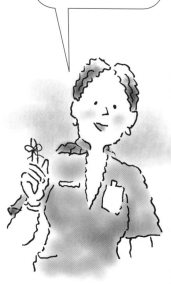

Remember that every patient may have different needs. The nursing diagnoses listed here are those that are most commonly associated with each medical condition.

- Risk of acute confusion related to hepatic encephalopathy syndrome
- Risk of imbalanced fluid volume related to ascites
- Risk of infection related to liver disease

Liver transplantation

- Acute pain related to surgery
- Compromised family coping related to prolonged disease
- Inadequate nutritional intake related to:
  - anorexia
  - chronic illness
  - initial postoperative nil-by-mouth status
- Ineffective breathing pattern related to prolonged general anesthesia and a large abdominal incision
- Anxiety related to fear of organ rejection
- Risk of deficient fluid volume related to high-dose steroid therapy and fluid loss
- Risk of impaired liver function related to surgery and disease process
- Risk of infection related to surgical incision and immunosuppression

Lung abscess

- Hyperthermia related to infection
- Impaired gas exchange related to altered oxygen supply
- Ineffective airway clearance related to increased secretions

Lung cancer

- Activity intolerance related to imbalance between oxygen supply and demand
- Inadequate nutritional intake related to inability to ingest food
- Ineffective airway clearance related to fatigue
- Powerlessness related to perceived mortality

Lupus erythematosus

- Decreased cardiac output related to pericarditis, myocarditis or endocarditis
- Hyperthermia related to immunosuppression
- Impaired physical mobility related to joint inflammation
- Impaired skin integrity related to rashes
- Risk-prone health behaviour related to disability

Lyme disease

- Acute pain related to arthritis
- Anxiety related to long treatment course
- Fatigue related to infection
- Impaired skin integrity related to rash

Lymphoma, non-Hodgkin's

- Anxiety related to unknown hospital procedures and threat to health status
- Lack of knowledge about self care related to lack of exposure to information
- Altered body image related to effects of chemotherapy or radiation therapy
- Inadequate nutritional intake related to:
  - altered oral mucous membrane
  - anorexia
  - fatigue
  - nausea and vomiting
  - taste alterations
- Impaired skin integrity related to effects of radiation therapy
- Ineffective protection related to immunosuppression
- Risk of infection related to:
  - chemotherapy
  - leucopoenia, lymphopenia from bone marrow involvement
  - radiation therapy effects

Macular degeneration

- Altered sensory perception (visual) related to aging process
- Impaired physical mobility related to vision impairment
- Powerlessness related to illness progression

Malignant melanoma

- Altered body image related to skin lesion
- Impaired skin integrity related to sore, inflamed, itchy skin lesion
- Anxiety related to long-term prognosis

Mastectomy

- Anxiety related to fear of cancer recurrence
- Lack of knowledge about treatment options related to lack of exposure to information
- Altered body image related to loss of a body part
- Risk of infection related to incision

Mechanical ventilation

- Inability to independently maintain activities of daily living related to impaired mobility status
- Deficient fluid volume related to:
  - altered oral intake
  - fluid retention
  - osmotic diuresis

- Fear related to inability to speak and dependence on life support
- Inadequate nutritional intake related to inability to ingest nutrients orally or digest them satisfactorily
- Impaired bed mobility related to ventilator
- Impaired gas exchange related to insufficient oxygen levels
- Ineffective airway clearance related to:
  - increased secretions
  - presence of an endotracheal tube
  - underlying disease
- Risk of impaired skin integrity related to physical immobility
- Risk of infection related to central venous catheter
- Risk of injury related to:
  - complications of invasive devices
  - bypassed safety alarm mechanisms
  - increased intrathoracic pressure
  - mechanical breakdown
  - patient deterioration

Ménière's disease

- Lack of knowledge about symptom prevention and control measures related to recent onset of disease
- Altered sensory perception (auditory, kinesthetic) related to disease process
- Impaired physical mobility related to vertigo

Meningitis

- Acute pain related to headache, joint involvement, muscle aches from infection
- Hyperthermia related to infection
- Ineffective tissue perfusion (cerebral) related to increased intracranial pressure
- Risk of injury related to seizures

Metabolic acidosis

- Acute confusion related to increased body acid
- Deficient fluid volume related to active loss from diarrhoea and vomiting
- Ineffective breathing pattern related to fatigue and Kussmaul's respirations
- Nausea related to GI distress

Metabolic alkalosis

- Altered thought processes related to acid–base imbalance
- Ineffective breathing pattern related to hypoventilation
- Risk of injury related to muscle weakness

Motor neurone disease

- Caregiver role strain related to complexity of care needs
- Impaired physical mobility related to muscular atrophy
- Impaired spontaneous ventilation related to respiratory muscle loss of enervation
- Impaired swallowing related to neuromuscular impairment
- Ineffective airway clearance related to retained secretions
- Inability to independently maintain normal activities related to lack of gross and fine motor skills

Multiple myeloma

- Acute pain related to neoplasm that infiltrates the bone
- Fatigue related to illness
- Risk of infection related to immunosuppression

Multiple sclerosis

- Compromised family coping related to effects of progressive, debilitating disease on family members and resultant alteration in role-related behaviour patterns
- Constipation related to decreased peristalsis
- Dressing/grooming self-care deficit related to neuromuscular impairment
- Fatigue related to weakness and spasticity
- Impaired physical mobility related to demyelinisation
- Impaired verbal communication related to dysarthria
- Interrupted family processes related to role disturbance and uncertain future
- Powerlessness related to remissions and exacerbations of illness
- Risk of injury related to:
  - gait impairment
  - vertigo
  - vision disturbances
- Altered sexual function related to fatigue, decreased sensation, muscle spasm or urinary incontinence
- Situational low self-esteem related to progressive, debilitating effects of disease
- Urinary retention related to sensorimotor deficits

Myasthenia gravis

- Activity intolerance related to muscle fatigue and weakness
- Inability to independently maintain activities of daily living related to neuromuscular involvement
- Fatigue related to muscle weakness
- Impaired swallowing related to cerebella dysfunction

- Ineffective airway clearance related to impaired ability to cough
- Ineffective therapeutic regime management related to insufficient knowledge of disease
- Risk of injury related to vision disturbance and weakness
- Risk of spiritual distress related to chronic illness
- Risk of urge urinary incontinence related to neuromuscular involvement

Myocardial infarction

- Activity intolerance related to weakness and fatigue
- Acute pain (chest) related to decreased myocardial oxygenation
- Fear of dying related to diagnosis
- Decreased cardiac output related to altered heart rate, rhythm
- Lack of knowledge about diagnostic procedures, therapeutic interventions and long-range implications for lifestyle changes related to complex diagnosis and therapeutic regime
- Impaired gas exchange related to ventilation–perfusion imbalance
- Ineffective coping related to fear of death, anxiety, denial or depression
- Risk of constipation related to diet, bed rest or medications
- Risk of injury related to myocardial ischemia, injury, necrosis, inflammation or arrhythmias

Myocarditis

- Activity intolerance related to weakness and fatigue
- Decreased cardiac output related to arrhythmias
- Fatigue related to infection

Nephrectomy

- Acute pain related to surgical procedure
- Ineffective airway clearance related to:
  – anesthesia
  – immobility
  – location of incision
  – pain
  – presence of chest tube
- Risk of imbalanced fluid volume related to decreased renal reserve and third-space fluid shifting immediately after surgery
- Risk of perioperative positioning related to flank positioning and outermost arm positioning

Nephrotic syndrome

- Inadequate nutritional intake related to high-protein, low-sodium diet
- Risk of imbalanced fluid volume related to disease process
- Risk of infection related to immunosuppression

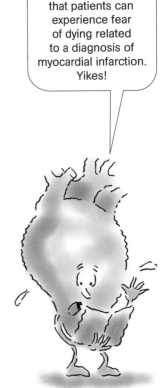

Says here that patients can experience fear of dying related to a diagnosis of myocardial infarction. Yikes!

Neuritis, peripheral

- Altered sensory perception (tactile) related to degeneration of peripheral nerves
- Impaired physical mobility related to muscle weakness
- Risk of injury related to disturbed sensory perception

Neurogenic bladder

- Reflex urinary incontinence related to neuromuscular dysfunction of the lower urinary tract
- Risk of compromised human dignity related to incontinence
- Risk of infection related to incomplete emptying of bladder

Obesity

- Activity intolerance related to excessive energy demands secondary to obesity
- Altered body image related to social stigma of obesity
- Inadequate nutritional intake related to:
  - dysfunctional eating patterns
  - energy expenditure imbalance
  - excess food intake
  - inherited disposition
  - sedentary activity level
- Impaired gas exchange related to ventilation–perfusion imbalance
- Impaired physical mobility related to fatigue with minimal exertion, joint or back discomfort, limitation of motion from extra skin folds
- Ineffective management of weight related to lack of knowledge
- Risk of impaired skin integrity related to:
  - altered circulation (oedema)
  - multiple moist skin folds
  - nutritional deficit

Oesophageal cancer

- Acute pain related to:
  - fistula
  - surgery
  - tumour
- Fatigue related to cachexia
- Inadequate nutritional intake related to dysphasia
- Risk of aspiration related to dysphasia

Oesophageal diverticula

- Inadequate nutritional intake related to dysphasia and regurgitation
- Risk of aspiration related to dysphasia and regurgitation
- Risk of infection related to inadequate primary defences

Osteoarthritis

- Activity intolerance related to pain
- Chronic pain related to deterioration of joint cartilage
- Impaired coping at home related to inadequate support systems, decreased range of motion with increased joint pain

Osteomyelitis

- Acute pain related to inflammation
- Lack of knowledge about prolonged treatment regime for infection and measures to prevent recurrence related to new diagnosis
- Impaired physical mobility related to pain
- Risk of anxiety related to prolonged infection, pain and immobilization
- Risk of injury related to use of antibiotics with high potential for toxic side effects

Osteoporosis

- Anxiety related to change in health status
- Altered body image related to joint deformity
- Altered patterns of sexual activity related to pain
- Risk of trauma related to bone loss

Otosclerosis

- Lack of knowledge about the disease related to lack of exposure to information
- Altered sensory perception (auditory) related to decreased motion of bones of the middle ear
- Risk of infection related to surgery

Ovarian cancer

- Constipation related to GI obstruction
- Inadequate knowledge about the disease and treatment options related to lack of exposure to information
- Grieving related to potential loss
- Urinary retention related to obstruction

Ovarian cyst

- Acute pain related to complications of ovarian cysts that cause acute abdominal symptoms
- Anxiety related to laparoscopic surgery
- Altered sexual patterns related to irregular or prolonged bleeding

Paget's disease

- Acute pain related to impingement of abnormal bone on spinal cord
- Inability to independently maintain activities of daily living related to musculoskeletal impairment
- Altered body image related to musculoskeletal impairment
- Impaired physical mobility related to asymmetrical bowing of tibia and femur

Pancreatic cancer

- Acute pain related to tumour pressure
- Anxiety related to threat of death and disease status
- Caregiver role strain related to illness severity
- Inadequate nutritional intake related to:
  - impaired digestion
  - loss of appetite
  - pain
  - vomiting

Pancreatitis

- Acute pain related to:
  - abscess formation or haemorrhaging
  - autodigestive processes and necrosis
  - oedema of the pancreas and surrounding tissues
  - peritonitis
- Inadequate nutritional intake related to:
  - gastric suction
  - impaired digestion
  - nil-by-mouth status
  - vomiting
- Nausea related to gastric distension
- Risk of deficient fluid volume related to:
  - fluid shifts
  - haemorrhage
  - hyperglycaemia
  - vomiting
- Risk of infection related to trauma and chronic disease
- Risk of injury related to:
  - alcoholism
  - hypovolemia
  - pulmonary insults

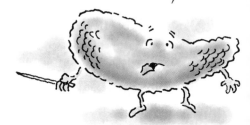

Watch patients with pancreatitis for signs of imbalanced nutrition. I'm feeling queasy just looking at this list.

Parkinson's disease

- Activity intolerance related to neuromuscular impairment
- Inability to independently maintain activities of daily living related to neuromuscular impairment

- Impaired coping at home related to disease effects
- Risk of aspiration related to impaired muscles of swallowing
- Risk of falls related to impaired gait and balance

Pelvic inflammatory disease

- Acute pain related to inflammation
- Risk of infection related to inadequate primary defences
- Altered patterns of sexual activity related to malaise and profuse, purulent vaginal discharge

Peptic ulcers

- Acute pain related to ulcers
- Lack of knowledge about ulcer prevention and care related to the need for long-term management
- Nausea related to GI distress

Percutaneous transluminal coronary angioplasty

- Acute pain related to restrictions on mobility and percutaneous puncture at groin site
- Anxiety related to known risks associated with the procedure
- Lack of knowledge about postdischarge care related to lack of exposure to information
- Risk of injury related to break in skin and presence of foreign body intravascularly

Pericarditis

- Acute pain related to inflammation of pericardium
- Decreased cardiac output related to pericarditis
- Ineffective tissue perfusion (cardiopulmonary) related to decreased cellular exchange

Peripheral vascular disease

- Activity intolerance related to pain
- Impaired physical mobility related to pain and activity intolerance
- Impaired tissue integrity (peripheral) related to decreased oxygenation
- Risk of peripheral neurovascular dysfunction related to vascular obstruction

Perirectal abscess and fistula

- Acute pain related to abscess and fistula
- Delayed surgical recovery related to inflammation
- Situational low self-esteem related to difficult healing process

Peritonitis

- Acute pain related to inflammation
- Nausea related to increased GI pressure
- Risk of infection related to inadequate primary defences

Permanent pacemaker insertion

- Inability to independently maintain activities of daily living related to bed rest and activity limitations
- Lack of knowledge about self-care after discharge related to unfamiliar therapeutic intervention
- Altered body image related to dependence on pacemaker
- Risk of infection related to surgical disruption of skin barrier

Pituitary tumour

- Acute pain related to tumour pressure
- Lack of knowledge about surgical options related to lack of exposure to information
- Altered sensory perception (visual) related to unilateral blindness
- Risk of injury related to dementia

Pleural effusion and emphysema

- Fatigue related to weakness
- Hyperthermia related to infection
- Ineffective breathing pattern related to pain and increased work of breathing

Pleurisy

- Acute pain related to inflammation of visceral and parietal pleurae
- Impaired gas exchange related to altered oxygen supply
- Ineffective breathing pattern related limited movement on affected side

Pneumocystis carinii pneumonia

- Fatigue related to infection
- Grieving related to poor prognosis
- Ineffective breathing pattern related to fatigue
- Risk of imbalanced body temperature related to infection

Pneumonia

- Acute pain related to fever and pleuritic irritation
- Inability to independently maintain activities of daily living related to weakness and tiredness
- Deficient fluid volume related to active fluid volume loss

- Inadequate knowledge about treatment regime related to lack of exposure to information
- Impaired gas exchange related to ventilation–perfusion imbalance
- Ineffective airway clearance related to retained secretions
- Risk of infection related to stress and other risk factors

Pneumothorax

- Acute pain related to air trapped in the intrapleural space
- Fear related to sudden onset of illness
- Impaired gas exchange related to ventilation–perfusion imbalance
- Ineffective tissue perfusion (cardiopulmonary) related to collapsed lung

Polycystic kidney disease

- Acute pain related to kidney mass
- Lack of knowledge about illness related to lack of exposure to information
- Ineffective tissue perfusion (renal) related to kidney mass

Polycythemia vera

- Acute pain related to headache
- Inadequate knowledge about disease and treatment related to lack of exposure to information
- Altered sensory perception (visual) related to hypervolemia
- Impaired gas exchange related to dyspnoea

Potassium imbalance

- Decreased cardiac output related to arrhythmias
- Diarrhoea related to hypercalcaemia and hypocalcaemia
- Nausea related to GI distress

Pressure ulcers

- Inadequate nutritional intake related to inability to digest and absorb nutrients
- Impaired physical mobility related to musculoskeletal and neuromuscular impairment
- Impaired skin integrity related to:
  - altered circulation
  - altered sensation
  - impaired physical mobility
  - mechanical factors
- Risk of infection related to impaired skin integrity

Prostatectomy

- Acute pain related to:
  - bladder spasms

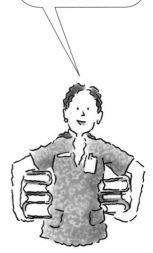

Lack of exposure to information can lead to deficient knowledge about an illness. I thought I might do a little reading about polycystic kidney disease.

    – catheter obstruction
    – surgical intervention
    – urethral stricture
- Risk of deficient fluid volume related to prostatic or incisional bleeding after surgery
- Risk of infection (postoperative) related to:
  - abdominal drain placement
  - preoperative status
  - urinary catheter
- Risk of low self-esteem related to:
  - incontinence
  - potential impotence
  - altered patterns of sexual activity
- Altered sexual function (decreased libido) related to:
  - decreased self-esteem
  - fear of incontinence
  - impotence related to parasympathetic nerve damage (from radical prostatectomy)
  - infertility related to retrograde ejaculation (from transurethral resection of the prostate and suprapubic prostatectomy)
- Urge urinary incontinence related to:
  - decrease in detrusor muscle
  - sphincter tone
  - trauma to the bladder neck
  - urinary catheter removal
- Urinary retention related to urinary catheter obstruction

Prostatic cancer

- Acute pain related to physical, biological or chemical agents
- Anxiety related to change in health status
- Altered sexual function related to impotence
- Urinary retention related to obstruction

Prostatitis

- Acute pain related to infection and destruction of tissue
- Hyperthermia related to infection
- Impaired urinary elimination related to infection

Psoriasis

- Altered body image related to itchy, dry, cracked and encrusted lesions on body parts
- Impaired skin integrity related to itchy, dry, cracked and encrusted lesions
- Social isolation related to disturbed body image

Pulmonary oedema

- Decreased cardiac output related to tachycardia
- Dysfunctional ventilatory weaning response related to anxiety
- Excess fluid volume related to fluid accumulation in extra vascular spaces of the lungs
- Ineffective breathing pattern related to diminished lung compliance

Pulmonary embolism and infarction

- Activity intolerance related to imbalance between oxygen supply and demand
- Acute pain related to biological injury
- Compromised family coping related to potentially life-threatening situation
- Decreased cardiac output related to altered heart rate and rhythm
- Deficient fluid volume related to active fluid volume loss
- Lack of knowledge about treatment regime related to complex disorder and therapy
- Impaired gas exchange related to ventilation–perfusion mismatch

Pulmonary hypertension

- Inability to independently maintain activities of daily living related to fatigue
- Decreased cardiac output related to altered heart rate and rhythm
- Ineffective breathing pattern related to hypertrophy of small pulmonary arteries
- Ineffective tissue perfusion (cardiopulmonary) related to impaired transport of oxygen across alveolar and capillary membranes

Pyelonephritis

- Excess fluid volume related to compromised regulatory mechanisms
- Hyperthermia related to infection
- Impaired urinary elimination related to urgency, burning or nocturia
- Risk of infection related to inadequate primary and secondary defences

Radioactive implant for cervical cancer

- Altered patterns of sexual activity related to vaginal tissue changes or fear of radioactivity
- Risk of complications related to imposed bed rest
- Risk of injury related to dislodgment of the implant

Raynaud's disease

- Altered sensory perception (tactile) related to decreased oxygenation
- Ineffective tissue perfusion (peripheral) related to decreased arterial blood flow
- Risk of impaired skin integrity related to decreased sensation and ischemia

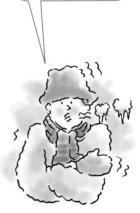

Patients with Raynaud's disease are at risk for impaired skin integrity related to decreased sensation. Is it cold in here, or is it just me?

Renal calculi

- Acute pain related to obstruction of ureter or kidney by renal calculi
- Lack of knowledge (disease) related to lack of exposure to information
- Risk of infection related to trauma
- Urinary retention related to ureter obstruction by renal calculi

Renal dialysis

- Acute pain related to haemodialysis treatment
- Inadequate nutritional intake related to:
  - abdominal distension
  - anorexia
  - nausea
  - stomatitis
- Impaired physical mobility related to lengthy treatment regime
- Ineffective breathing pattern related to elevation of diaphragm during peritoneal dialysis exchanges and reduced mobility
- Risk of acute confusion related to consequences of long-term dialysis treatment
- Risk of fluid imbalance related to dialysis
- Risk of infection related to invasive procedure
- Risk of injury related to:
  - bleeding from the area around the vascular access device
  - potential for thrombosis, stenosis or haematoma of vascular access
- Risk of injury (perforation or ileus) related to catheter insertion or irritation from dialysate

Renal failure, acute

- Inadequate knowledge about acute renal failure and dialysis related to lack of exposure to information on complex disease and its management
- Excess fluid volume related to sodium and water retention
- Inadequate nutritional intake related to anorexia, nausea and vomiting and restricted dietary intake
- Impaired urinary elimination related to disease process
- Risk of infection related to decreased immune response and skin changes secondary to uraemia
- Risk of injury related to uremic syndrome

Renal failure, chronic

- Caregiver role strain related to illness chronicity
- Chronic low self-esteem related to chronic disease
- Altered thought processes related to:
  - acidosis
  - fluid and electrolyte imbalances
  - uremic toxins

- Excess fluid volume related to fluid retention
- Inadequate nutritional intake related to:
  - altered metabolism of proteins, lipids and carbohydrates
  - anorexia
  - diarrhoea
  - GI inflammation with poor absorption
  - nausea and vomiting
  - restricted dietary intake
- Impaired oral mucous membrane related to accumulation of urea and ammonia
- Nonconcordance with treatment regime related to:
  - deficient knowledge
  - denial
  - lack of resources
  - lack of social support systems
- Risk of impaired skin integrity related to:
  - abnormal blood clotting
  - anaemia
  - calcium phosphate deposits on the skin
  - capillary fragility
  - decreased activity of oil and sweat glands
  - retention of pigments
  - scratching
- Altered sexual function related to the effects of uraemia on the endocrine system and central nervous system and to the psychosocial impact of chronic renal failure and its treatment

Respiratory acidosis

- Decreased cardiac output related to altered heart rate and rhythm
- Impaired gas exchange related to ventilatory–perfusion imbalance
- Ineffective breathing pattern related to hypoventilation

Respiratory alkalosis

- Anxiety related to hyperventilation
- Impaired gas exchange related to ventilatory–perfusion imbalance
- Ineffective breathing pattern related to hyperventilation

Retinal detachment

- Altered sensory perception (visual) related to loosening of retina
- Impaired physical mobility related to vision disturbance
- Ineffective coping related to decreased vision and impending surgery

Rheumatoid arthritis

- Activity intolerance related to pain and swelling of joints
- Chronic pain related to inflammation of joints

- Altered body image related to arthritic joints
- Anxiety regarding loss of independence related to lack of mobility

Salmonella

- Diarrhoea related to GI distress
- Hyperthermia related to infection
- Risk of deficient fluid volume related to diarrhoea

Sarcoidosis

- Activity intolerance related to pain
- Decreased cardiac output related to arrhythmias
- Lack of knowledge about disease and treatment related to lack of exposure to information
- Ineffective breathing pattern related to pain

Scabies

- Impaired skin integrity related to skin infection
- Altered patterns of sexual activity related to fear of spreading infection
- Social isolation related to fear of spreading infection

Seizures

- Acute confusion related to postictal state
- Lack of knowledge about seizure management related to the need to maintain safety
- Impaired memory related to neurological disturbance
- Ineffective airway clearance related to:
  - airway occlusion by tongue or foreign body
  - apnoea
  - excessive secretions
  - jaw clenching
  - loss of consciousness
- Risk of injury related to excessive uncontrolled muscle activity
- Risk of trauma related to internal factors

Septic shock

- Acute confusion related to decreased cerebral tissue perfusion
- Diarrhoea related to GI irritation
- Hyperthermia related to infection
- Inadequate nutritional intake related to inadequate intake and active fluid and nutrient loss
- Impaired gas exchange related to ventilation–perfusion imbalance and diffusion defects
- Ineffective coping related to threat to life
- Risk of injury due to complications related to ischemia or bleeding

Sinusitis

- Acute pain related to inflammation and pressure
- Fatigue related to infection
- Risk of infection related to inadequate primary defences

Sjögren's syndrome

- Altered sensory perception (visual) related to ocular dryness
- Fatigue related to disease process
- Impaired oral mucous membrane related to oral dryness

Skin grafts

- Lack of knowledge about care of donor and graft sites related to the need for follow-up care after discharge
- Altered body image related to wound and potential scarring
- Inadequate nutritional intake related to increased metabolic needs secondary to tissue healing
- Impaired physical mobility related to position and movement limitations
- Risk of infection of donor site related to surgical excision

Spinal cord injury

- Inability to independently maintain activities of daily living related to spinal cord injury
- Constipation related to loss of voluntary bowel control
- Decreased cardiac output related to autonomic dysfunction and immobility
- Inability to engage in usual hobbies and activities related to loss of mobility or function
- Altered body image related to physical disability
- Inadequate nutritional intake related to acute injury
- Impaired gas exchange related to loss of use of phrenic nerve, intercostal muscles or abdominal muscles secondary to the spinal injury
- Impaired coping at home related to inadequate support systems
- Impaired physical mobility related to muscular paralysis
- Impaired urinary elimination related to interruption of neural innervation
- Incontinence, bowel and total urinary related to neuromuscular enervation
- Ineffective airway clearance related to loss of use of intercostal muscles
- Risk of autonomic dysreflexia related to damage to spinal cord with another associated stressor
- Risk of infection related to catheterisation

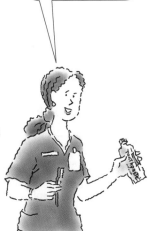

Spinal cord injuries can cause many deficits related to self-care. Brush up on the ones listed here.

Spinal neoplasm

- Impaired physical mobility related to neuromuscular impairment
- Incontinence, bowel and total urinary related to neurological dysfunction

- Risk of autonomic dysreflexia related to spinal cord injury or lesion
- Risk of impaired skin integrity related to:
  - altered nutritional status
  - altered sensation
  - mechanical factors
  - moisture from incontinence
  - physical immobilisation

Squamous cell carcinoma

- Anxiety related to threat to health status
- Impaired skin integrity related to invasive tumour of skin
- Ineffective therapeutic regime management related to deficient knowledge

Stroke

- Inability to independently maintain activities of daily living related to:
  - neuromuscular impairment
  - perceptual cognitive impairment
  - weakness or lack of motivation
- Caregiver role strain related to increased care needs
- Chronic confusion related to cerebral injury
- Lack of knowledge about stroke management related to lack of exposure to information on long-term care
- Impaired physical mobility related to damage to motor cortex or motor pathways
- Impaired verbal communication related to cerebral injury
- Ineffective airway clearance related to hemiplegic effects of a stroke
- Ineffective tissue perfusion (cerebral) related to clot or haemorrhage
- Risk of disuse syndrome related to neuromuscular impairment
- Unilateral neglect related to cerebral injury

Syphilis

- Ineffective coping related to situational crisis
- Altered sexual patterns related to fear of spreading illness
- Risk of infection related to external factors

Tendonitis and bursitis

- Activity intolerance related to pain and stiffness
- Acute pain related to inflammation
- Inability to engage in normal activities related to restricted movement of joint due to pain

Thoracotomy

- Acute pain related to surgical incision
- Lack of knowledge about treatment regime related to unfamiliarity with thoracotomy

- Impaired gas exchange related to:
  - analgesic medications
  - atelectasis
  - hypoventilation from anaesthesia
  - pain
  - thickened secretions
- Risk of infection related to surgical incision and endotracheal intubation

Thrombocytopenia

- Decreased cardiac output related to tachycardia
- Inadequate knowledge about disease and treatment related to lack of exposure to information
- Fatigue related to disease process
- Risk of injury related to possible bleeding from lack of platelets

Thrombophlebitis

- Acute pain related to vessel obstruction and oedema
- Inadequate knowledge about treatment regime related to lack of exposure to information
- Ineffective tissue perfusion (peripheral) related to interruption of venous flow

Thyroid cancer

- Inadequate knowledge about treatment regime related to lack of exposure to information
- Impaired swallowing related to pressure of thyroid nodule
- Ineffective breathing pattern related to enlarged thyroid nodule

Toxic shock syndrome

- Diarrhoea related to infection
- Fear related to sudden onset of illness
- Hyperthermia related to infection

Tracheotomy

- Impaired skin integrity related to humidity, moisture or mucus accumulation
- Ineffective breathing pattern related to tracheal tube dislodgment or plugging
- Risk of aspiration related to impaired swallowing and vomiting
- Risk of injury (poor oxygenation) related to suctioning procedure

Trauma

- Impaired gas exchange related to:
  - head injury

- – pulmonary injury
- – shock
- Impaired physical mobility related to orthopaedic injury
- Risk of imbalanced fluid volume related to hypovolemia or cardiac injury
- Risk of injury (complications) related to:
  - – hyper metabolic state
  - – impaired immunologic defences
  - – stress
- Risk of post-trauma syndrome related to perception of event and sudden, unexpected injury

Trigeminal neuralgia

- Acute pain related to disorder of the fifth cranial nerve
- Anxiety related to threat to health
- Ineffective coping related to inadequate level of perception of control

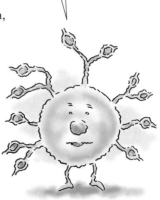

Trigeminal neuralgia can cause acute pain. What nerve!

Tuberculosis

- Inadequate knowledge about disease process related to lack of exposure to information
- Ineffective airway clearance related to tracheobronchial obstruction or secretions
- Ineffective breathing pattern related to decreased energy or fatigue
- Risk of infection related to altered primary defences
- Social isolation related to fear of spreading disease

Ulcerative colitis

- Anxiety related to change in health status
- Diarrhoea related to inflammation of colon
- Fatigue related to loss of fluids and diarrhoea
- Inadequate nutritional intake: less than body requirements related to inability to absorb nutrients
- Inability to perform normal activities of daily living related to frequent diarrhoea

Urinary tract infection

- Acute pain related to inflammation and muscle spasms
- Inadequate knowledge about disease process related to lack of exposure to information
- Risk of confusion related to infection
- Impaired urinary elimination related to obstruction

Urolithiasis

- Acute pain related to:
  - – incision

– passage of calculus fragments
– procedural manipulation
• Lack of knowledge about potential causes of calculus formation related to new diagnosis
• Impaired urinary elimination: dysuria, oliguria, pyuria or frequency related to:
– calculus fragment passage
– haematuria
– infection
– obstruction

Uterine cancer

• Acute pain related to cancer
• Inadequate nutritional intake related to cancer
• Spiritual distress related to chronic illness

Uterine prolapse

• Anxiety related to change in health status
• Altered body image related to biophysical factors
• Stress urinary incontinence related to weak pelvic musculature

Valvular heart disease

• Activity intolerance related to fatigue and dyspnoea on exertion
• Anxiety related to change in health status
• Decreased cardiac output related to mechanical disruption
• Ineffective breathing pattern related to decreased energy and fatigue

Vascular retinopathy

• Altered sensory perception (visual) related to disturbed blood supply to the eye
• Ineffective coping related to chronic illness
• Risk of injury related to loss of vision

Vasculitis

• Altered body image related to illness
• Inadequate nutritional intake related to anorexia of disease process
• Ineffective tissue perfusion (cerebral, cardiopulmonary, GI, renal, peripheral) related to inflamed vessels causing impaired blood flow to nearby organs
• Risk of infection related to impaired defences

Vulvovaginitis

• Acute pain related to inflammation
• Altered sexual function related to vaginal inflammation, itching and irritation
• Risk of infection related to inadequate primary defences

Wounds

- Acute pain related to trauma to nerve endings
- Impaired skin integrity related to penetration of skin
- Risk of contamination related to detrimental home environmental factors
- Risk of deficient fluid volume related to active loss from trauma
- Risk of infection related to inadequate primary defences

Just the facts

In this chapter, you'll learn:

♦ nursing diagnoses that correlate with common maternal–neonatal medical diagnoses.

A look at maternal–neonatal diagnoses

This chapter covers medical diagnoses that are applicable to pregnant patients and their neonates. Maternal–neonatal care can be complex because both the mother and neonate have many needs. The diagnoses listed here are just a sampling of the diagnoses that you might encounter on a maternity unit. Each entry provides a list of a few of the major nursing diagnoses and related factors to be considered after your assessment. Remember that the nursing diagnoses listed here represent the needs most commonly associated with the medical condition; your patient may have different needs related to other activities of daily living.

> Maternal–neonatal care must address the needs of both the mother and the neonate.

Abortion

- Anxiety related to situational crisis or unmet needs
- Complicated grieving related to loss of foetus
- Risk of deficient fluid volume related to bleeding

Abruptio placenta

- Acute pain related to separation of placenta
- Deficient fluid volume related to bleeding

- Grieving related to potential loss of foetus
- Ineffective tissue perfusion (cardiopulmonary of neonate) related to decreased cellular exchange

Acquired immunodeficiency syndrome—Infant

- Fear (parent) related to infant's future death as a result of human immunodeficiency virus (HIV) infection
- Risk of infection related to perinatal transmission of HIV and immunosuppression
- Risk of injury related to transmission of HIV to personnel and other infants in the nursery

Cardiovascular disease in pregnancy

- Activity intolerance related to heart failure
- Decreased cardiac output related to heart decompensation and arrhythmias
- Risk of imbalanced fluid volume related to compromised regulatory mechanism

Caesarean birth

- Activity intolerance related to:
  - anaesthetic administration
  - delivery
  - pain
  - surgical incision
- Acute pain related to surgical incision
- Ineffective coping related to surgical intervention, perceived loss of the birthing experience and fatigue
- Risk of deficient fluid volume related to bleeding associated with surgery
- Risk of infection (maternal) related surgical incision, repeated vaginal examination, sequelae of anaesthetic administration, bladder intubation or I.V. lines

Choanal atresia

- Ineffective family coping related to:
  - anxiety
  - emotional conflict as a result of infant's defect
  - guilt
- Ineffective breathing pattern related to obstruction from congenital defect

Diabetes-related complications during pregnancy

- Inadequate nutritional intake related to altered carbohydrate metabolism
- Ineffective breathing pattern related to uterine enlargement and excessive amniotic fluid
- Risk of infection related to disease process
- Risk of injury (foetal) related to dependence on maternal glycemic states

Two diabetes-related complications associated with ineffective breathing patterns are uterine enlargement and excessive amniotic fluid.

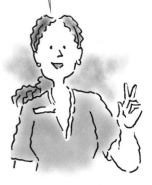

Drug addiction and withdrawal

• Lack of knowledge about safe, healthy neonatal care and development related to emotional inadequacy and lack of exposure to information about infant care
• Inadequate nutritional intake related to:
– poor or low intake because of lack of coordination in sucking or swallowing
– vomiting
• Ineffective coping (maternal) related to drug abuse or inability to care for the infant
• Ineffective infant feeding pattern related to delayed neurological development
• Risk of deficient fluid volume related to diarrhoea or vomiting
• Risk of impaired skin integrity related to perianal irritation from diarrhoea and rubbing against sheets because of hyperactivity
• Risk of injury (respiratory and neurological) related to withdrawal from drug exposure

Ectopic pregnancy

• Acute pain related to disruption of pelvic tissue
• Deficient fluid volume related to bleeding
• Fear related to loss of pregnancy and threat to fertility
• Risk of infection related to the trauma of tubal rupture and peritoneal inflammation

Foetal alcohol syndrome

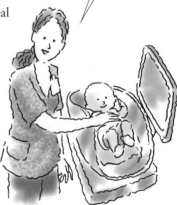

Foetal alcohol syndrome can cause delays in growth and development.

• Lack of knowledge about safe parenting related to lack of information about infant care
• Delayed growth and development related to neurological and mental deficiency
• Altered family relationships related to abuse of alcohol
• Inadequate nutritional intake related to lack of nutritional reserves and to poor intake
• Risk of impaired parenting related to previous lifestyle associated with alcohol abuse or to unrealistic expectations of self and infant

Hydrocephalus

• Anxiety (parent and child) related to lack of understanding about the child's condition and treatment
• Compromised family coping related to illness of baby
• Delayed growth and development related to disease
• Excess fluid volume related to placement of ventriculoatrial shunt
• Inadequate nutritional intake related to feeding difficulties
• Ineffective tissue perfusion (cerebral) related to increased intracranial pressure

- Risk of deficient fluid volume related to altered nutritional status in the preoperative and postoperative phases
- Risk of infection related to surgical placement of shunt
- Risk of injury related to onset of seizures

Hyperemesis gravidarum

- Acute pain related to repeated episodes of vomiting
- Deficient fluid volume related to protracted emesis
- Fear related to hospitalisation and pregnancy outcome
- Inadequate nutritional intake related to nausea and vomiting and subsequent inconsistent or insufficient food intake

Hypertension, pregnancy-induced

- Lack of knowledge about signs and symptoms of increased blood pressure related to lack of exposure to information
- Excess fluid volume related to compromised regulatory mechanism
- Risk of injury (foetal) related to impaired maternal–placental perfusion
- Risk of injury (maternal) related to organ or system dysfunction as a sequela of vasospasm and increased blood pressure

Hysterectomy

- Acute pain related to abdominal incision and distension
- Altered body image related to changes in body appearance and function as a result of surgery
- Altered sexual function related to:
  – altered body image
  – concerns about acceptance by spouse or partner
  – decreased oestrogen levels
  – fatigue
  – grieving
  – loss of vaginal sensations
  – pain
  – sexual activity restrictions
- Urinary retention related to decreased bladder and urethral muscle tone from anaesthesia and mechanical trauma

Mastitis and breast engorgement

- Acute pain related to inflammation and milk engorgement
- Risk of imbalanced body temperature related to infection
- Risk of infection related to inadequate primary defences

Meconium aspiration syndrome

- Impaired family coping related to anxiety and guilt
- Ineffective breathing pattern related to meconium aspiration

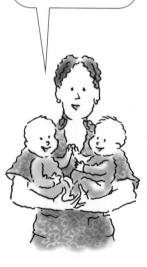

A dramatic increase in family size can lead to ineffective coping. Sure, these two can be a handful, but imagine trying to juggle quadruplets.

Multiple gestation

- Ineffective coping related to dramatic increase in family size
- Risk of injury (maternal and foetal) related to physiological demands of a multiple pregnancy
- Risk of injury related to preterm labour and delivery

Myelomeningocele

- Constipation related to level of spinal cord injury
- Delayed growth and development related to the hospital stay
- Hypothermia related to heat loss through the sac
- Inadequate nutritional intake related to surgery
- Impaired skin integrity related to presence of sac and surgical procedure
- Impaired urinary elimination related to injury of spinal cord nerves
- Ineffective tissue perfusion (cerebral) related to hydrocephalus and increased intracranial pressure
- Risk of impaired parenting related to separation from the infant at birth
- Risk of impaired skin integrity related to contact with urine or faeces and altered mobility

Necrotising enterocolitis

- Diarrhoea related to inflammation
- Ineffective infant feeding pattern related to nil-by-mouth status
- Altered family dynamics related to shift in health status of family member

Neural tube defects

- Anxiety regarding decision (possible abortion) related to genetic defect
- Altered family dynamics related to change in health status of family member
- Spiritual distress related to chronic illness

Placenta previa

- Anxiety related to unknown hospital procedures
- Deficient fluid volume related to active loss, bleeding
- Fear related to unknown foetal outcome
- Risk of injury (foetal) related to uteroplacental insufficiency

Premature rupture of membranes

- Anxiety related to situational crisis
- Risk of infection related to lack of primary defences

Puerperal infection

- Acute pain related to inflammatory processes and exudate entrapment
- Anxiety related to threat to health status
- Risk of infection related to the trauma of labour, delivery and the iatrogenic introduction of pathogens

Respiratory distress syndrome

- Decreased cardiac output related to disease
- Impaired family coping related to anxiety, guilt and separation from the infant as a result of situational crisis
- Inadequate nutritional intake related to:
  - decreased gastric motility
  - inability to ingest feedings
  - withholding of food and water
- Impaired gas exchange related to:
  - alveolar ventilation
  - lung perfusion
  - reduced lung volume and compliance
- Risk of deficient fluid volume related to active fluid losses
- Risk of injury related to medical therapy and treatments

Toxoplasmosis

- Lack of knowledge of effective treatment regimes related to lack of exposure to information
- Fatigue related to localised infection
- Hyperthermia related to infection

10 Children's diagnoses

Just the facts

In this chapter, you'll learn:

♦ nursing diagnoses that correlate with common children's medical diagnoses.

A look at children's diagnoses

This chapter covers medical diagnoses that are common in children. Remember that children can have the same medical and nursing diagnoses as adults; however, the care provided for these patients may be different. Each entry provides a list of a few of the major nursing diagnoses and related factors to be considered after your assessment. Remember that the nursing diagnoses listed here represent the needs most commonly associated with the medical condition in children; your patient may have different needs.

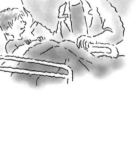

Although children can have the same diagnoses as adults, the care provided may be different.

Acne vulgaris

- Lack of knowledge about skin care related to lack of exposure to information
- Low self-esteem related to face lesions
- Social isolation related to alteration in physical appearance

Anorexia nervosa

- Deficient fluid volume related to active loss
- Altered body image related to psychological effects of the disorder
- Inadequate nutritional intake related to fear of obesity
- Impaired social interaction related to low self-esteem
- Altered family relationships related to illness of family member
- Social isolation related to eating habits

Aplastic and hypoplastic anaemias

- Fatigue related to disease process
- Ineffective breathing pattern related to weakness and fatigue
- Ineffective family coping related to altered health status of family member
- Risk of infection related to destruction of stem cells in bone marrow

Asthma

- Activity intolerance related to imbalance between oxygen supply and demand
- Anxiety related to threat to health status
- Lack of knowledge about how to manage asthma related to new diagnosis
- Lack of knowledge about effective treatment regimes related to lack of previous experience
- Fatigue related to hypoxia
- Impaired gas exchange related to bronchial constriction
- Ineffective airway clearance related to constriction
- Risk of deficient fluid volume related to loss of fluid from the respiratory tract

Attention deficit hyperactivity disorder

- Impaired social interaction related to hyperactivity
- Altered family dynamics related to shift in health status of family member
- Risk of delayed development related to brain disorder

Autistic disorder

- Impaired social interaction related to brain disorder
- Impaired verbal communication related to stimulus confusion
- Risk of impaired parenting related to 24-hour demands of child with special needs
- Risk of other-directed or self-directed violence related to impaired capacity to identify and express feelings

Biliary atresia

- Deficient fluid volume related to poor absorption of nutrients
- Lack of knowledge about biliary atresia related to new diagnosis
- Delayed growth and development related to chronic illness

Bronchiolitis

- Anxiety (child and parent) related to lack of knowledge about condition
- Lack of knowledge about home care procedures related to new diagnosis
- Fatigue related to respiratory distress
- Hyperthermia related to infection

- Inadequate nutritional intake related to increased metabolic needs
- Impaired gas exchange related to bronchiolar oedema and increased mucus production
- Risk of deficient fluid volume related to increased water loss through exhalation and decreased fluid intake
- Social isolation related to isolation precautions

Bronchopulmonary dysplasia

- Anxiety (parent) related to fear and lack of knowledge about the child's illness
- Delayed growth and development related to chronic illness, prematurity or prolonged hospital stay
- Inadequate nutritional intake related to increased metabolic rate and high calorie demands
- Impaired gas exchange related to atelectasis
- Risk of impaired parenting related to chronic illness
- Risk of impaired skin integrity related to irritation from nasogastric tube feedings

Bulimia nervosa

- Constipation related to poor eating habits and insufficient fluid intake
- Deficient fluid volume related to active loss
- Altered body image related to illness
- Altered personal identity related to body weight
- Inadequate nutritional intake related to binge-purge behaviour

Cerebral palsy

- Inability to maintain own activities of daily living related to involuntary movements and impaired muscle function
- Caregiver role strain related to complex needs of care receiver
- Delayed growth and development related to neuromuscular impairment
- Impaired physical mobility related to impaired muscle function
- Impaired swallowing related to impaired muscle function

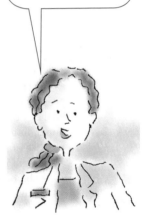

Involuntary movements and impaired muscle function associated with cerebral palsy can lead to deficits in self-care skills.

Child abuse

- Delayed growth and development related to inadequate care-giving
- Impaired parenting related to the abusive parent's inability to attach to or bond with the child
- Ineffective family coping related to personal issues that contribute to child abuse
- Risk of other-directed violence (abusive family member) related to maladaptive behaviour

Cleft lip and cleft palate

- Impaired family coping related to the stress of hospitalisation (preoperative)
- Inadequate nutritional intake related to impaired feeding (preoperative)
- Impaired skin integrity related to surgical incision
- Ineffective infant feeding pattern related to deformity
- Risk of aspiration related to ineffective feeding

Clubfoot

- Compromised family coping related to situational crisis
- Lack of knowledge about treatment protocol related to lack of exposure to information
- Impaired physical mobility related to casting or splinting
- Risk of impaired skin integrity related to casting or splinting
- Risk of injury related to failure to provide appropriate care, leading to complications

Congenital heart defect

- Anxiety (child) related to:
  - immobility
  - intensive care unit environment
  - parental anxiety
  - separation from parents
  - surgery
- Anxiety (parent) related to child's congenital heart defect
- Decreased cardiac output related to disease process and surgical procedure
- Lack of knowledge about preoperative and postoperative care related to impending surgery
- Risk of infection related to immobility and numerous incisions
- Risk of injury related to:
  - blood loss
  - electric current
  - positioning
  - surgical procedure

Congenital hip dysplasia

- Constipation related to immobility
- Inability to engage in normal activities (boredom) related to immobility secondary to traction or spica cast
- Risk of impaired skin integrity related to:
  - immobility
  - spica cast
  - traction

• Risk of infection related to break in skin integrity secondary to traction (if pins are used)
• Risk of injury related to possible mechanical malfunctioning of traction or circulatory compromise

Croup

- Anxiety related to hospital stay and respiratory distress
- Ineffective airway clearance related to laryngeal obstruction
- Ineffective breathing pattern related to upper airway oedema and thickened secretions
- Risk of deficient fluid volume related to decreased oral intake
- Risk of infection related to break in primary defences

Cystic fibrosis

- Anxiety (child) related to respiratory distress and hospital stay
- Anxiety (parent) related to lack of knowledge about the child's condition
- Lack of knowledge about home care procedures related to complex disorder
- Inadequate nutritional intake related to reduced absorption of nutrients
- Impaired gas exchange related to increased mucus production
- Parental role conflict related to child's hospitalisation
- Risk of delayed development related to illness
- Risk of infection related to increased mucus production

Down's syndrome

- Bathing/hygiene, dressing/grooming self-care deficit related to developmental delay
- Altered family dynamics related to chronic illness
- Risk of delayed development related to chromosome abnormality

Epiglottiditis

- Anxiety (parent) related to lack of knowledge concerning the child's condition
- Anxiety and fear (child) related to respiratory distress and hospital stay
- Impaired family coping related to anxiety and fear
- Hyperthermia related to infection
- Impaired swallowing related to inflammation and oedema
- Ineffective airway clearance related to inflammation and oedema
- Ineffective breathing pattern related to upper airway oedema
- Risk of deficient fluid volume related to decreased fluid intake

Fracture

- Bathing/hygiene, dressing/grooming, feeding self-care deficit related to immobility of affected limb

- Impaired mobility related to cast or splints
- Risk of injury related to inability to use body part
- Acute pain related to muscle spasm, swelling or bleeding
- Constipation related to immobility
- Impaired gas exchange related to complications secondary to the fracture and immobility
- Ineffective tissue perfusion (peripheral) related to:
  – bleeding
  – swelling
  – the cast
  – traction
- Risk of boredom related to immobility from cast or traction
- Risk of impaired skin integrity related to immobility from cast or traction

Fragile X syndrome

- Delayed growth and development related to X-linked dominant gene inheritance
- Impaired verbal communication related to mental retardation
- Interrupted family processes related to shift in health status of family member
- Risk of caregiver role strain related to complex care needs of care receiver

Glycogen storage disease

- Anxiety (parent) related to lack of knowledge concerning the child's condition
- Delayed growth and development related to chronic illness
- Readiness for enhanced nutrition related to readiness to manage disease through diet

Haemophilus influenza infection

- Deficient fluid volume related to active loss
- Hyperthermia related to infection
- Impaired gas exchange related to ventilation–perfusion imbalance

Head injury

- Acute pain related to head injury
- Anxiety (child and parent) related to traumatic head injury
- Decreased cardiac output related to haemorrhage
- Lack of knowledge about follow-up monitoring related to lack of information given
- Ineffective breathing pattern (with potential for respiratory failure) related to increased intracranial pressure (ICP)
- Ineffective tissue perfusion (peripheral) related to hypotension secondary to hypovolemic shock
- Risk of deficient fluid volume related to nausea and vomiting

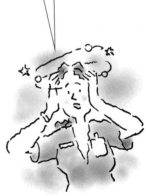

Traumatic head injury can cause anxiety for both the child and the parent. What if my head never stops spinning?

- Risk of impaired skin integrity related to physical immobility
- Risk of infection related to injury
- Risk of injury related to altered level of consciousness secondary to head injury or increased ICP (or both)
- Risk of injury secondary to seizures

Haemophilia

- Acute pain related to bleeding and swelling
- Chronic low self-esteem related to chronic illness and hospital stay
- Compromised family coping related to repeated hospital stays and the child's chronic illness
- Impaired physical mobility related to decreased range of motion secondary to bleeding and swelling
- Risk of injury (haemorrhage) related to disease

Hirschsprung's disease

- Anxiety (parent) related to lack of knowledge about the disease and prescribed treatment
- Constipation related to aganglionosis
- Altered body image related to colostomy or ileostomy
- Impaired skin integrity related to exposure to stools secondary to colostomy or ileostomy
- Risk of deficient fluid volume related to:
  - decreased intake
  - increased absorptive surface of distended bowel
  - nausea and vomiting
- Risk of infection of incision related to contamination from stools

Hypopituitarism

- Anxiety related to treatment regime
- Risk of delayed development related to deficiency of anterior pituitary hormones
- Risk of disproportionate growth related to deficiency of anterior pituitary hormones

Hypospadias and epispadias

- Acute pain related to surgery
- Anxiety (child and parent) related to surgical procedure (urethroplasty)
- Risk of infection (urinary tract) related to placement of indwelling catheter
- Risk of injury related to dislodged urinary catheter or urinary catheter removal

Impetigo

- Lack of knowledge about treatment and prevention of recurrence of infection related to new diagnosis

- Impaired skin integrity related to skin infection
- Risk of infection related to inadequate primary defences

Intraventricular haemorrhage

- Lack of knowledge about infant's condition and potential for home care related to the new injury
- Risk of injury related to fragility of the capillary beds in the cerebrum

Intussusception

- Acute pain related to bowel strangulation
- Anxiety (parent) related to surgery
- Nausea related to vomiting

Juvenile rheumatoid arthritis

- Chronic pain related to joint inflammation
- Altered body image related to the effects of the chronic illness and the disabling nature of the disease
- Impaired physical mobility related to joint inflammation
- Impaired skin integrity related to immobility
- Risk of imbalanced body temperature related to disease process

Kyphosis

- Altered body image related to altered physical appearance
- Risk of situational low self-esteem related to altered physical appearance

Leukaemia, acute

- Hopelessness related to illness
- Ineffective protection related to immunosuppression
- Risk of imbalanced body temperature related to infection
- Risk of infection related to altered primary and secondary defences

Mononucleosis

- Fatigue related to weakness
- Altered family dynamics related to family member becoming temporary full-time caregiver
- Risk of imbalanced body temperature related to infection

Mumps

- Acute pain related to inflammation
- Fatigue related to infection
- Hyperthermia related to infection

Muscular dystrophy

- Caregiver role strain related to increased care needs
- Dressing/grooming, feeding self-care deficit related to muscle weakness and disability
- Impaired physical mobility related to muscle weakness
- Ineffective health maintenance related to inability to care for self

Myringotomy

- Anxiety (child and parent) related to the surgical procedure and perioperative events
- Lack of knowledge about home care procedures related to new treatment
- Risk of injury (haemorrhage) related to surgery

Osteomyelitis

- Chronic pain related to inflammation and infection
- Compromised family coping related to prolonged hospital stay
- Inadequate nutritional intake related to increased metabolic needs for wound healing
- Impaired physical mobility related to infection
- Impaired skin integrity related to infection
- Risk of infection related to wound contamination

Otitis media

- Acute pain related to inflammation of the middle ear
- Altered sensory perception (auditory) related to complications of otitis media
- Risk of infection related to impaired primary defences

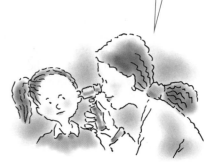

Some children with otitis media experience acute pain related to inflammation.

Pediculosis

- Impaired skin integrity related to itching and redness
- Low self-esteem related to lice
- Social isolation related to feelings of embarrassment due to diagnosis

Phenylketonuria

- Altered thought processes related to delayed mental development
- Impaired skin integrity related to dry skin lesions
- Risk of delayed development related to accumulation of phenylalanine in blood

Pyloric stenosis

- Acute pain related to surgical incision
- Anxiety (parent) related to lack of understanding about the disease, diagnostic studies and treatment
- Deficient fluid volume related to dehydration or shock (or both)
- Inadequate nutritional intake related to frequent projectile vomiting
- Risk of infection related to surgery

Respiratory syncytial virus infection

- Inadequate nutritional intake: less than body requirements related to inability to ingest foods
- Ineffective breathing pattern related to decreased energy
- Risk of deficient fluid volume related to active loss and inflamed mucous membranes of the throat

Reye's syndrome

- Anxiety and fear (child) related to hospital stay
- Decreased intracranial adaptive capacity related to decreased cerebral perfusion
- Ineffective breathing pattern (with the potential for respiratory failure) related to cerebral oedema
- Ineffective thermoregulation related to illness
- Ineffective tissue perfusion (cardiopulmonary, cerebral, renal) related to ICP
- Ineffective tissue perfusion (cerebral) related to increased ICP and cerebral oedema
- Risk of impaired parenting related to the child's hospital stay or lack of knowledge about the child's condition
- Risk of impaired skin integrity related to physical immobility
- Risk of injury (hypoglycaemia) related to decreased calorie intake or possible metabolic dysfunction or both

Rheumatic fever and rheumatic heart disease

- Acute pain related to joint pain
- Decreased cardiac output related to carditis
- Hyperthermia related to infection

Roseola infantum

- Lack of knowledge about child's care needs and prognosis related to new diagnosis
- Hyperthermia related to infection
- Impaired skin integrity related to skin rash

Rubella

- Lack of knowledge about child's care needs and prognosis related to new diagnosis
- Hyperthermia related to infection
- Impaired skin integrity related to skin rash

Rubeola

- Fatigue related to disease
- Hyperthermia related to infection
- Impaired skin integrity related to pruritic rash

Scoliosis

- Acute pain related to curvature of spine
- Altered body image related to altered body shape
- Risk of impaired skin integrity related to brace

Sickle cell anaemia

- Acute pain related to vascular occlusion and tissue hypoxia
- Deficient fluid volume related to decreased fluid intake and the kidneys' inability to concentrate urine
- Impaired gas exchange related to decreased oxygen-carrying capacity of blood
- Ineffective tissue perfusion (peripheral) related to blood vessel obstruction secondary to sickling of red blood cells

Spinal cord defects

- Lack of knowledge about spinal cord defects related to lack of exposure to information
- Delayed growth and development related to spinal cord defect
- Disabled family coping related to increased care giving demands on family with minimal social support

Tay–Sachs disease

- Delayed growth and development related to muscle weakness
- Disabled family coping related to family member with unexpressed feelings of anxiety
- Grieving related to death of child

Tonsillitis

- Acute pain related to throat swelling
- Hyperthermia related to infection
- Impaired swallowing related to swelling

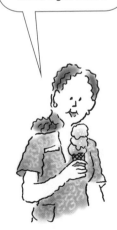

Tonsillitis can cause pain and difficulty swallowing. Luckily, ice cream slides right down!

Tracheoesophageal fistula

- Anxiety (parent) related to lack of knowledge about the disorder, diagnostic testing and treatment
- Delayed growth and development related to the hospital stay and deprivation of normal parent-infant interactions and environmental stimulation
- Ineffective airway clearance related to aspiration of secretions or feedings or both
- Ineffective breathing pattern related to choking, coughing and cyanosis during feeding

Tympanoplasty

- Anxiety (child and parent) related to surgical procedure and perioperative events
- Risk of injury (haemorrhage) related to surgery

Varicella

- Acute pain related to rash
- Impaired skin integrity related to itchy rash
- Interrupted family processes related to family member having to stay home from work to care for child

11 Mental health diagnoses

Just the facts

In this chapter, you'll learn:

♦ nursing diagnoses that correlate with common mental health medical diagnoses.

A look at mental health diagnoses

This chapter covers common mental health medical diagnoses. Each entry provides a list of a few of the major nursing diagnoses and related factors to be considered after your assessment of a patient with the particular medical diagnosis. Remember that the nursing diagnoses listed here represent the needs most commonly associated with the medical condition; your patient may have different needs.

Abusive disorders, sexual or physical

- Dysfunctional family processes related to violence
- Post-trauma syndrome related to:
  - interpersonal violence
  - physical neglect or abuse
  - sexual abuse or assault
- Risk of compromised human dignity related to abuse.

Addictive disorders

Alcohol dependence
- Anxiety related to:
  - alcohol withdrawal
  - poor self-concept
  - real or perceived threats to physical safety

- Chronic low self-esteem related to:
  - coping difficulties
  - guilt
  - shame about alcohol abuse
  - unmet expectations
- Altered sensory perception (visual, auditory, tactile) related to acute alcohol withdrawal
- Dysfunctional family processes: alcoholism related to role disruptions caused by the patient's alcohol-related disorder
- Inadequate nutritional intake related to:
  - effects of chronic alcohol intake on digestive organs
  - interference of alcohol in absorption and metabolism of nutrients
  - poor dietary intake while consuming alcohol
- Insomnia related to alcohol abuse and decreased rapid eye movement sleep cycle
- Risk of injury related to:
  - alcohol withdrawal
  - depression
  - seizures
  - suicidal thoughts
- Risk-prone health behaviour related to alcohol abuse

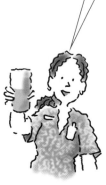

Alcohol dependence can lead to risk for injury related to withdrawal, depression, seizures and suicidal ideation. Another reason to stay addicted to water. Cheers!

Hallucinogenic substance abuse

- Altered sensory perception (visual, auditory, kinesthetic, gustatory, tactile, olfactory) related to decreased cognitive function resulting from hallucinogen intake
- Altered thought processes related to:
  - hallucinogen abuse as evidenced by auditory or visual hallucinations
  - impaired memory
  - inattentiveness
  - problem-solving inabilities
- Insomnia related to hallucinogen abuse or intoxication as evidenced by verbal complaints of sleeping inability, nightmares or interrupted sleep
- Risk of injury related to impaired judgement and disorientation
- Risk of injury related to poisoning by use of adulterated street drugs
- Risk-prone health behaviour related to substance abuse

Polysubstance abuse

- Chronic low self-esteem related to perceived failures and lack of positive feedback
- Altered sensory perception (visual, auditory, tactile) related to multiple psychoactive substance withdrawal
- Ineffective coping related to maladaptive reliance on alcohol and other drugs
- Powerlessness related to lack of control over psychoactive substance use

Stimulant abuse
- Decreased cardiac output related to stimulant use
- Lack of knowledge about the risks of stimulant abuse related to denial of need for information
- Altered sensory perception (visual, auditory, kinesthetic) related to sensory overload from stimulant use
- Fear related to altered thought processes
- Inadequate nutritional intake related to placing greater importance on drug use than on eating
- Impaired social interaction related to isolation associated with drug use
- Insomnia related to stimulant use
- Risk of imbalanced body temperature related to stimulant use
- Risk of impaired skin integrity related to changes in health maintenance
- Risk of other-directed violence related to:
  - difficulty processing and interpreting thoughts
  - sensory overload from stimulant use
- Risk-prone health behaviour related to substance abuse

Substance abuse (sedatives, opioids)
- Lack of knowledge about the risks of substance abuse related to inability to process or retain information while impaired and in denial
- Ineffective denial related to feelings of low self-esteem
- Risk of infection related to:
  - compromised immunity
  - high-risk behaviours
  - insufficient knowledge about disease
- Risk-prone health behaviour related to substance abuse

Adjustment disorder
- Complicated grieving related to:
  - inhibited grieving
  - multiple losses and bereavement processes
- Defensive coping related to:
  - inadequate support systems
  - personal vulnerability
  - unmet expectations
  - work overload
- Impaired social interaction related to decreased perception of appropriate social behaviour
- Risk-prone health behaviour related to:
  - disability requiring lifestyle changes
  - impaired cognition
  - inadequate support systems
  - unresolved grieving

Anxiety disorder

- Anxiety related to:
  - stresses in home or work environments, close interpersonal relationships
  - threat to self-concept
  - unmet needs
- Chronic low self-esteem related to lack of positive feelings and difficulty concentrating
- Risk of inadequate nutritional intake: less than body requirements related to inability to ingest food due to psychological factors
- Social isolation related to panic state

Bipolar disorder

- Chronic low self-esteem related to depressive state and feelings of hopelessness, need to continue long-term medications
- Altered thought processes related to mood swings from mania to depression
- Impaired home maintenance related to difficulty concentrating and flight of ideas
- Sleep deprivation related to manic state

Delusional disorder

- Altered thought processes related to false beliefs that are based in reality
- Impaired social interaction related to delusional behaviour
- Social isolation related to delusional behaviour

Depression

- Chronic low self-esteem related to stress or loss
- Deficient diversional activity related to lack of interest
- Altered body image related to illness
- Inadequate nutritional intake related to poor eating habits
- Ineffective coping related to obsessive negative thoughts and feelings
- Risk of caregiver role strain related to psychological needs of care receiver
- Risk of loneliness related to self-imposed social isolation
- Risk of self-directed violence related to self-help
- Social isolation related to inability to engage in satisfying personal relationships

Dissociative disorder

- Disturbed personal identity related to underdeveloped ego, threat to self-concept or childhood abuse or trauma
- Ineffective coping related to a severe level of repressed anxiety
- Interrupted family processes related to shift in health status of family member

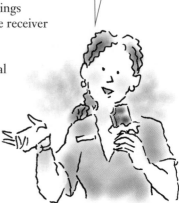

Preoccupation with eating behaviours or rituals can lead to impaired social interaction.

Eating disorders

- Lack of knowledge about nutrition and eating disorders related to lack of interest in learning and denial of condition
- Altered body image related to misperceived physical appearance
- Inadequate nutritional intake: less than body requirements related to refusal to eat, purging activities or excessive physical exercise
- Impaired social interaction related to withdrawal from peer group, fear of rejection and preoccupation with eating behaviours or rituals
- Ineffective denial related to a lack of knowledge about real or potential dangers associated with eating disorders
- Interrupted family processes related to a perfectionist, overprotective or chaotic family system
- Risk of injury related to excessive exercise or potentially harmful behaviours

Gender identity disorder

- Anxiety related to conflict between desires and expected sex role behaviour
- Altered personal identity related to conflict between anatomical sex and gender identity
- Altered sexual patterns related to conflicts with sexual orientation
- Interrupted family processes related to family confusion and anxiety about gender of family member

Panic disorder

- Anxiety related to panic disorder
- Chronic low self-esteem related to repeated episodes of apprehension and fear
- Post-trauma syndrome related to perception of event or sudden loss

Personality disorder–Cluster A

- Impaired social interaction related to disorganized thinking, odd or eccentric behaviours, emotional coldness
- Ineffective coping related to:
  - inability to trust others
  - self-absorption
  - unusual perceptions and communication patterns
- Interrupted family processes related to shift in health status of family member

Personality disorder–Cluster B

- Impaired social interaction related to:
  - behaviours that produce hostility in others
  - inability to form healthy interpersonal relationships
  - low self-esteem

- Ineffective coping related to:
  - fear of abandonment
  - feelings of loneliness, emptiness, boredom
  - poor frustration tolerance
  - poor impulse control
- Risk of other-directed or self-directed violence related to dramatic, emotional or erratic behaviour or low self-esteem

Personality disorder—Cluster C

- Anxiety related to preoccupation
- Altered thought processes related to indecision or doubt over decisions
- Ineffective coping related to:
  - need to always be right and perfect
  - need to use rules and routines to maintain a secure environment
  - the inability to ask for help
  - verbal manipulation
- Interrupted family processes related to rigidity in functions, roles and rules
- Powerlessness related to:
  - intellectualisation or denial of feelings as a means to gain self-control
  - perfectionist behaviour that protects against inferiority feelings
- Sleep deprivation related to prolonged psychological discomfort
- Social isolation related to an inability to establish and maintain relationships

Phobias

- Altered personal identity related to inability to control fear
- Fear related to anxiety about an object or situation
- Ineffective coping related to persistent irrational fear

Post-traumatic stress disorder

- Hopelessness related to feelings of helplessness and loss of control
- Post-trauma syndrome related to traumatic event
- Powerlessness related to uncertainty about the future

Schizophrenia

- Anxiety related to disturbance in thought content
- Bathing/hygiene self-care deficit related to apathy and delusions
- Caregiver role strain related to chronic illness
- Disturbed thought processes related to genetic, biochemical, psychological and socio-cultural causes

Sleep disorder

- Anxiety related to inability to sleep
- Insomnia related to:
  - external factors, such as hospital routines, environmental noise and changing work shifts

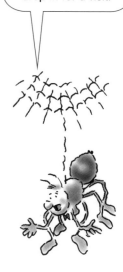

Persistent irrational fear can lead to ineffective coping. Stand back, folks. I'm about to drop in for a visit.

- medical illness
- pain
- psychological stress
- Interrupted family processes related to family member not being able to fulfil role requirements because of lack of sleep

Somatoform and factitious disorders

- Bathing/hygiene, dressing/grooming self-care deficit related to:
  - activity intolerance
  - neuromuscular or musculoskeletal impairment
  - pain or discomfort
  - perceptual or cognitive impairment
- Caregiver role strain related to unpredictable illness and conflict with care receiver
- Chronic pain related to unmet dependency needs or repressed anxiety as demonstrated by verbal complaints with no pathophysiological validation
- Lack of knowledge about healthy social interactions related to:
  - denial
  - intense repressed anxiety level
  - lack of interest in learning
  - preoccupation with self and pain
- Impaired family coping related to struggle for control and power
- Altered body image related to low self-esteem evidenced by preoccupation with real or imagined altered body structure or function
- Ineffective coping related to:
  - extreme need for approval and acceptance
  - inability to manage emotional conflict
  - low self-esteem
  - unmet dependency needs
- Social isolation related to physical symptoms or disability

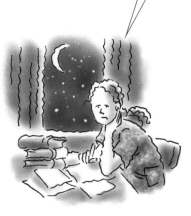

Patients with sleep disorders can experience anxiety-related inability to sleep. At this point, even the sheep have gone to sleep.

Vicarious traumatisation

- Insomnia related to recurrent nightmares or dreams of personal death and fear of their recurrence
- Post-trauma syndrome related to the subjective experience of single or multiple traumatic events through repeated exposure to trauma victims (vicarious traumatisation)
- Powerlessness related to:
  - inadequate problem-solving and coping skills
  - overwhelming anxiety

Appendices and index

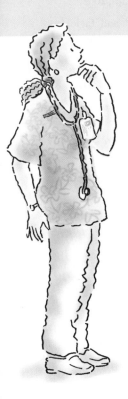

Selected references

British National Formulary, London: BMJ Publishing Group, 2006.

Carpenito-Moyet, L.J. *Nursing Care Plans & Documentation: Nursing Diagnosis and Collaborative Problems*, 4th ed. Philadelphia: Lippincott Williams & Wilkins, 2004.

Carpenito-Moyet, L.J. *Understanding the Nursing Process: Concept Mapping and Care Planning for Students.* Philadelphia: Lippincott Williams & Wilkins, 2007.

Ignatavicius, D., and Workman, M.L. *Medical-Surgical Nursing: Critical Thinking for Collaborative Care*, 5th ed. Philadelphia: W.B. Saunders Co., 2006.

Johnson, M., et al. *NANDA, NOC, and NIC Linkages*, 2nd ed. Philadelphia: Mosby, 2006.

Klossner, N.J. *Introductory Maternity Nursing.* Philadelphia: Lippincott Williams & Wilkins, 2006.

McCloskey-Dochterman, J., and Bulechek, G., eds. *Nursing Interventions Classification (NIC)*, 4th ed. St. Louis: Mosby, 2004.

Moorehead, S., et al., eds. *Iowa Outcomes Project: Nursing Outcomes Classification (NOC)*, 3rd ed. St. Louis: Mosby, 2004.

Nursing and Midwifery Council. *Standards for Medicine Management*, London: Nursing and Midwifery Council, 2007.

Nursing and Midiwfery Council. *The Code: Standards of Conduct, Performance and Ethics for Nurses and Midwives*, London: Nursing and Midwifery Council, 2008.

Nursing Student Success Made Incredibly Easy. Philadelphia: Lippincott Williams & Wilkins, 2005.

Pearson, A., et al., *Nursing Models for Practice*, 3rd ed. Edinburgh: Butterworth Heinemann, 2005.

Shives, L. *Concepts of Psychiatric-Mental Health Nursing*, 7th ed. Philadelphia: Lippincott Williams & Wilkins, 2007.

Smeltzer, S. *Brunner and Suddarth's Textbook of Medical-Surgical Nursing*, 11th ed. Philadelphia: Lippincott Williams & Wilkins, 2007.

Sparks-Ralph, S., and Taylor, C. *Sparks and Taylor's Nursing Diagnosis Reference Manual*, 6th ed. Philadelphia: Lippincott Williams & Wilkins, 2005.

Wong, D., et al. *Maternal Child Nursing Care*, 3rd ed. Philadelphia: Mosby, 2006.

Integrated Care Pathway (Example)

Peterborough and Stamford Hospitals **NHS**
NHS Foundation Trust

**Cardiac Chest Pain (Acute Coronary Syndrome/Myocardial Infarction)
Integrated Clinical Pathway**

NHS NO:	Date of Admission: Time:
Patient No: Name:	Admission Ward: CCU 1Z
	Admitting Consultant:
Address:	Source A/E ☐ GP ☐ Paramedic ☐ Ward ☐
Patient telephone No:	**Reason for admission:**
Is this your permanent address? Y ☐ N ☐ Where have you been living in the last 12 months?	Baseline observations
	Temp °C Pulse /min Blood glucose mmol
If UK – evidence of right to live here seen? Y ☐ N ☐ OSV form completed – Date: Sign: If not UK, contact stage 2 officer or duty manager out of hours. Date / time : Sign:	Resps /min B/P mmHg O2 Sats %
	Urinalysis: *affix printout or document abnormalities*
Age Sex: M F D.O.B ____/____/____	
Married☐ Single☐ Widowed☐	
Separated☐ Divorced☐ Other☐	
Next of kin: Relationship: Address:	MSU/CSU required ☐ Sent date/time:
☎ Home: ☎ Work:	Past Medical History:
First contact: Relationship:	
☎ Home: ☎ Work:	Initial ECG changes and Rhythm:
Other ☎ No's	**Final Diagnosis:**
NOK aware of Admission. Yes☐ No☐ With pt☐	Thrombolysis: Yes No Type:
Contact anytime Yes☐ No☐ Comments:	Cardiac blood tests:

Name of GP: Practice:	Date			
	Troponin			
Occupation	Cholesterol		Triglycerides	
Religion	MRSA Status			
	Positive ☐ Negative ☐ Screened ☐			
Ethnic group				
Language Interpreter Y / N Required	Unknown ☐ Prev Pos ☐ Date :_____			

Predicted discharge date (transfer info from page no. 6)			
PDD	Amended date:	Amended date:	Amended date:

Speech difficulties	Yes ☐	No ☐	
Comments			

Good hearing	Yes ☐		No ☐
Wears aids	Yes ☐	L R	No ☐
With pt on admission	Yes ☐		No ☐
Comments			

Good vision	Yes ☐	No ☐
Wears glasses	Yes ☐	No ☐
Contact Lenses	Yes ☐	No ☐
With pt on admission	Yes ☐	No ☐
Comments		

Has dentures	Yes ☐	No ☐
Top	Yes ☐	No ☐
Bottom	Yes ☐	No ☐
With pt on admission	Yes ☐	No ☐
Comments		

Sleep pattern   Good ☐   Fair ☐   Poor ☐

Aids to sleep?   Yes ☐   No ☐

Comments

Mental State

Pressure Areas Intact   Yes ☐   No ☐

Comments

Diet – Any Special Requirements?

How tall are you?

What is your normal **weight**?

Have you intentionally lost weight recently? Y ☐ N ☐
Have you been eating less than normal ? Y ☐ N ☐

If Yes to either of the above questions or BMI 19 or below, follow Nutrition Care plan

BMI =   = $\dfrac{\text{weight (kg)}}{\text{height (m)}^2}$

Personal Effects / Valuables:
Patients are strongly advised to hand over any money or valuables during their stay for safe custody. The Trust cannot accept any responsibility for any property not deposited in this manner.
Policy explained to patient by:
Signature:
Print name:

With patient   Yes ☐   No ☐
In safe/General Office Yes ☐
Date returned to patient:
Signature:
Print Name:
Property list completed   Yes ☐ No ☐

Micturition	Continent ☐	Incontinent ☐	
Bowels	Regular ☐	Irregular ☐	
Comments			

Fully Mobile	Yes ☐	No ☐
Walking Aids	Yes ☐	No ☐

Manual Handling Assessment required Yes ☐ No ☐
Falls assessment tool required   Yes ☐ No ☐
Bed rail assessment tool required Yes ☐ No ☐
Comments

Lives   Alone ☐   With others ☐

Lives in:
House	☐
Bungalow	☐
Flat	☐ Floor ☐
Residential	☐
Nursing Home	☐
Warden Controlled	☐
Comments	

Community Services   Comments:
Meals on wheels	☐
DN or CPN	☐
Home care	☐
Day care	☐
Social Worker	☐

Potential Discharge Problems?
Support care aware of admission? Yes ☐   No ☐

SSD Stage 1 ☐ Date:
SSD Stage 2 ☐ Date:

Stairs	☐ Comments:
Lift	
Toilet Up	☐
Toilet Down	☐
Bathroom Up	☐
Bathroom Down	☐

Contact details for MDT

Do you have an advanced direction/ Living Will?
Yes ☐   No ☐
If yes, ensure a copy is kept in the notes

Admitting Nurse

Ward:

Sign:

Print Name & Grade:

Date:

Clinical judgement should be used at all times

Peterborough and Stamford Hospitals
NHS Foundation Trust

Medical Assessment	Surname:
	First Name:
Presenting History	Unit No.
	Date of Birth:
Date & Time of onset of pain (include history and nature) + time of most severe pain	Or patient label

Past Medical History	
Details:	

Angina Yes ☐ No ☐

MI Yes ☐ No ☐

CABG Yes ☐ No ☐

Angio/PTCA Yes ☐ No ☐

Other conditions + Systems review:

TIMI risk score (on admission)	
Risk factor	**1 Point each**
Age ≥ 65	☐
≥3 CAD risk fx (FHx,HTN,↑Chol,DM,Smoker)	☐
Known CAD (Stenosis ≥50%) (previous MI/CABG/PCI)	☐
Aspirin use in past 7days	☐
Recent(<24 h) severe angina	☐
↑ Cardiac markers	☐
ST deviation ≥0.5 mm	
Total Risk score 0–7	☐
Low 0–2 ☐ Intermediate 3-4 ☐ High 5–7 ☐	

Risk Factors: ☐ ☐ **Details:**

Smoker Yes☐ No☐ Per day for .... years

Ex Smoker Yes☐ No☐ Gave up .... ago

Hypertension Yes☐ No ☐

Diabetes Mellitus Yes☐ No ☐

Family History Yes☐ No☐

Raised Cholesterol Yes☐ No ☐ Not Known ☐

Regular Medication & Doses:

Allergies:

Must also be documented in Alert notations Table on inside front cover of case note folder.

Peterborough and Stamford Hospitals **NHS**

NHS Foundation Trust

Cardiac Chest Pain/
Myocardial Infarction Pathway

Surname:	
First Name:	
Unit No.	
Date of Birth:	
Or patient label	

Clinical Examination Sheet

On examination:

CVS   Pulse   BP   JVP   HS

RS   **Abdomen**

O$_2$ Sats=   %   Resp rate:

CNS

GCS: Eyes [/ 4]   Verbal [/ 5]   Motor [/ 6]

Neurology grossly intact; not formally assessed [ ]

ECG & rhythm: **CXR:**

Consider primary angioplasty for **MI patients, or if ineligible, aim to commence thrombolysis within 20 minutes of patient's arrival in hospital**

Plan:- Investigations:		Treatment:	Impression:		
ECG x 3		Aspirin			
Urea/Electrolytes		Clopidogrel			
Glucose		Clexane	**Other interventions**		
Lipids		ACEI			
LFTS		BB			
FBC		Statin			
CXR		Thrombolysis			
			Print Name & Grade		
Troponin T after ...... am/pm		IV opiate			
		IV heparin	Drs Signature		
		IV nitrate	Bleep:	Date:	Time:

Date/Time	Registrar review	Signature/Name/Bp. No.

Date/Time	Post take consultant opinion

Resuscitation status   Not discussed ☐   For resus ☐   Discussed ☐   DNAR ☐   DNAR form completed ☐

PDD: (transfer date to page 1)

For further evaluation space go to page 8

Peterborough and Stamford Hospitals **NHS**
NHS Foundation Trust

**Cardiac Chest Pain/
Myocardial Infarction Pathway**

| Surname: |
| First Name: |
| Unit No. |
| Date of Birth: |
| Or patient label |

Goals of the ICP

Early and accurate diagnosis
Prompt and appropriate treatment
Prevention of complications
Secondary prevention – MI and related conditions
Return to usual lifestyle

Pain relief:

Oxygen	Up to 100% as required. Monitor O_2 saturations and pain level
Diamorphine	2.5–5 mg IV as required for moderate–severe pain. Drug of choice for AMI.
GTN*	1–2 tabs/puffs for mild ischaemic pain
Buccal GTN*	2–5 mg longer acting nitrate
ISDN IV*	2–10 mg/hr. Consider for recurrent pain. Monitor BP every 15 minutes initially

Treatment guidelines

Up-to-date **guidelines** are available as laminated **flowcharts** in all medical admission areas: CCU, MAU, AE and 2X Cardiology ward.
Full versions are accessible via the Intranet under the Cardiology department and within the clinical policies and guidelines.

The guidelines are:
- **Clinical guidelines for the use of Trop T measurement in the assessment of chest pain**
- **Clinical guidelines for the management of patients with acute myocardial infarction (STEMI)**
- **Clinical guidelines for the management of suspected acute coronary syndrome (includes management of ACS patients who are on warfarin)**
- **Clinical guidelines for the continuing care of patients with acute coronary syndrome or myocardial infarction**
- **Clinical guidelines for the management of patients with suspected or definite angina**

Latest **treatment guidelines** are also available at ward level (CCU, MAU, 2X) to guide prescribing for:

- STEMI (ST segment elevation Myocardial Infarction)
- NSTEMI (Non–ST segment elevation myocardial infarction) and ACS (acute coronary syndromes)

If in doubt about any of the guidelines or treatment choices please contact the Acute Coronary Syndrome Nurses on bleep 1744

* See abbreviation list on page No 12

Date/Time	Progress Notes & Variances – reason and action taken	Signature/Name/Bp. No.

Peterborough and Stamford Hospitals **NHS**
NHS Foundation Trust

Cardiac Chest Pain/
Myocardial Infarction Pathway

| Surname: |
| First Name: |
| Unit No. |
| Date of Birth: |
| Or patient label |

Date/Time	Progress Notes & Variances – reason and action taken	Signature/Name/Bp. No.

Add in further continuation sheets as necessary

Clinical judgement should be used at all times
MI ICP KW NOV 2000 REVISED Dec 2008 Review Dec 2013   Page 9 of 17

Peterborough and Stamford Hospitals
NHS Foundation Trust

Cardiac Chest Pain/ Myocardial Infarction Pathway

| Surname: |
| First Name: |
| Unit No. |
| Date of Birth: |
| Or patient label |

*delete as appropriate

Acute stage	Date:			
	N	E	L	N
ECG recording on admission and if pain recurs / change in condition				
Cardiac rhythm monitored				
IV Cannula checked for patency and flushed BD (use IV chart)				
O$_2$ % commenced as prescribed and monitor O$_2$ saturation				
Level of pain assessed on a scale of 0–10 and chart commenced				
Pain relief administered as per protocol and prescription				
Blood tests as requested + Trop T @ 12 hr (+ blood glucose strip-test for all patients)				
Baseline observations ⇨ progressively reduced until patient's condition stabilised				
$^1/_2$ hrly BP initially with IV nitrate infusion*				
Administer medications as prescribed				
If blood glucose >11.0 commence dextrose/insulin regime (see guideline)				
Patient orientated to CCU / Ward and reassured				
Carers aware of patient's condition, informed of visiting, Tel no. and care plan				
Bed rest maintained, up to the commode only				
Bed bath / assisted wash as required*				
Fluid balance chart maintained				
Nutrition-diet and fluids tolerated				
Pressure areas assessed – Waterlow score recorded				
Assess need for night sedation				
Assess if appropriate to progress to **Stage 1** level care				
Thrombolysis patients only:				
Administer Thrombolysis drugs as per protocol +/– IV Heparin*				
¼ hrly pulse / BP whilst receiving Thrombolysis				
ECG repeated 90 minutes after commencing thrombolysis				

Signatures, Name and Grade to be completed by Named Nurse for Shift

	Signature	Print Name	Print Grade
Night Duty			
AM			
PM			
Night Duty			

How to complete this legal document of care:

This document is **flexible** and any care not included can be added to show that all patients needs have been met.

Any variation from the pathway should be noted within the evaluation – document the code number, give a reason and any action taken.

Do **not** use ticks or crosses, except in the Yes/No boxes. **Initials, signatures and N/A** are the only accepted inscriptions.

Variance Codes					
Patient Condition		Staff		Department/Systems	
1	Pain Not Controlled	51	Doctor's Decision	101	Theatre Delay
2	Nausea & Vomiting	52	Doctor's Availability	102	Pharmacy Delay
3	Pyrexial (high temp)	53	Nurse's Decision	103	Transport Delay
4	Low temp	54	Nurse's Availability	104	Laboratory Delay
5	Hypertension (high bp)	55	Patient's Decision	105	X-ray Delay
6	Hypotension (low bp)	56	Patient's Availability	106	Community Care Availability
7	Oxygen Saturations below 95%	57	Family's Decision	107	Equipment Availability
8	Cannula removed	58	Family's Availability	108	Porter Delay
9	Confusion	59	Carer's Decision	109	Department Closed
10	Falls	60	Carer's Availability	110	Other
11	Arrhythmia	61		111	Bed unavailable on other ward
12	Heart failure	62		112	
13	Fluid balance continued	63		113	
50	MRSA	100		150	

References:

Department of Health (2000). National Service Frameworks. Coronary Heart Disease.
Heart attacks & other acute coronary syndromes.

British Cardiac Society Guidelines and Medical Practice Committee, and Royal College of Physicians Clinical Effectiveness and Evaluation Unit (2001). Guideline for the management of patients with acute coronary syndromes without persistent ECG ST segment elevation. Heart.

ESC. European Society of Cardiology-European Heart Journal (2002). Management of ACS in patients presenting without persistent ST-segment elevation.

Abbreviation List			
ACS	Acute Coronary Syndrome	MIBI	Isotope perfusion scan
AMI	Acute Myocardial Infarction	ACEI	Angiotensin-Converting Enzyme Inhibitor
BBB	Branch Bundle Block	GTN	Glyceryl Trinitrate
NSTEMI	Non-ST elevation Myocardial Infarction	ISDN	Isosorbide DiNitrate
SBP	Systolic blood pressure	GI	Gastro-intestinal
DBP	Diastolic blood pressure	CVA	Cerebral Vascular Accident
CCU	Coronary Care Unit	IV	Intravenous
STEMI	ST elevation Myocardial Infarction	MRSA	Methicillin-Resistant Staphylococcus-aureus

Peterborough and Stamford Hospitals **NHS**
NHS Foundation Trust

**Cardiac Chest Pain/
Myocardial Infarction Pathway**

*delete as appropriate

Surname:	
First Name:	
Unit No.	
Date of Birth:	
Or patient label	

Stage 1	Date:		
	E	L	N
Cardiac monitoring reviewed (discontinue after 24 hrs if stable)*			
Pain control assessed			
Provide bed bath or assisted wash*			
Gently walk out to the toilet (if pain free) or provide commodes/bottles*			
Sat out of bed as tolerated			
TDS observations recorded or as patient determines (see observation chart)			
IV cannula flushed with 0.9% Saline B/D (use IV chart) or consider removal*			
Serial ECG +/– ECG if pain recurs/change in condition			
Blood tests as required + Troponin T 12 hrs after cardiac event or worst pain			
Fluid balance chart reviewed (discontinued after 12 hrs if stable)*			
Nutritional needs met + assess bowel status (record on observation chart)			
Pressure areas assessed and Waterlow Score reassessed if ≥10			
Anxieties identified and discussed			
Assess need for night sedation			
Cardiac Rehabilitation Nurse Referral (on PAS) if applicable			
Relevant Rehabilitation / Information booklets given			
Patient to watch Angina or MI DVD if able			
Discuss care and progress with patient			
Patient ready to move from CCU to ward?*			
Assess if appropriate to progress to **Stage 2** level care			
Consider discharge if pain free + Troponin T level negative: commence **discharge checklist**			

Signatures, Name and Grade to be completed by Named Nurse for Shift			
	Signature	Print Name	Print Grade
Night Duty			
AM			
PM			
Night Duty			

Clinical judgement should be used at all times

Stage 1

Peterborough and Stamford Hospitals _NHS_
NHS Foundation Trust

Cardiac Chest Pain/ Myocardial Infarction Pathway

*delete as appropriate

| Surname: |
| First Name: |
| Unit No. |
| Date of Birth: |
| Or patient label |

Stage 2	Date:		
	E	L	N
Pain controlled			
Mobilised around the bed area and out to the toilet			
Encourage independence with wash or shower*			
At least one ½ hr rest period during the day			
TDS TPR and BP recorded if MI / ACS			
Serial ECG and copy given to patient			
Nutritional needs met			
IV cannula flushed or consider removal*			
Bowel status assessed			
Patient to watch Angina or MI DVD*			
Discuss care and progress with patient – **commence discharge planning**			
Consider discharge if pain free + Troponin T level negative: commence **discharge checklist**			
Assess if appropriate to progress to **Stage 3** level care			
Use this stage for patients transferred back from Papworth following PPCI			
Refer patient to Cardiac Rehabilitation team			
Inform ACS team of patients transfer back			

Signatures, Name and Grade to be completed by Named Nurse for Shift			
	Signature	**Print Name**	**Print Grade**
Night Duty			
AM			
PM			
Night Duty			

Stage 2

Peterborough and Stamford Hospitals

NHS Foundation Trust

**Cardiac Chest Pain/
Myocardial Infarction Pathway**

*delete as appropriate

| Surname: |
| First Name: |
| Unit No. |
| Date of Birth: |
| Or patient label |

Stage 3	Date:		
	E	L	N
Pain controlled			
Can mobilise around the ward without chest pain			
Stair Test Completed (AMI only)			
At least one ½ hr rest period during the day			
Twice a day TPR and BP recorded			
Anxieties identified and discussed			
Advice from Cardiac Rehabilitation / ACS nurse endorsed			
Washed in bathroom / shower*			
Bowel status assessed			
Nutritional needs met			
Discharge plans discussed – **commence checklist**			
Own Transport available for discharge Yes☐ No☐ if no refer to **discharge checklist**			
TTOs ordered (ensure GTN as TTO)			
Assess if appropriate for discharge → **Stage 4** level care			
Transfer to Papworth only:			
Commence Transfer to Papworth checklist			
Provide Papworth map / Cardiac Investigation information to patient and family			
Remain on **Stage 3** level care			
Bloods to be repeated every 5 days (minimum) prior to transfer – FBC and Creatinine/Electrolytes			

Signatures, Name and Grade to be completed by Named Nurse for Shift			
	Signature	Print Name	Print Grade
Night Duty			
AM			
PM			
Night Duty			

Stage 3

Peterborough and Stamford Hospitals

NHS Foundation Trust

**Cardiac Chest Pain/
Myocardial Infarction Pathway**

*delete as appropriate

| Surname: |
| First Name: |
| Unit No. |
| Date of Birth: |
| Or patient label |

Stage 4	Date:		
	E	L	N
Mobilising freely without chest pain			
At least one ½ hr rest period during the day			
Daily TPR and BP recorded			
Anxieties identified and discussed			
Advice from Cardiac Rehabilitation / ACS nurse endorsed			
Washed in bathroom / showered			
Nutritional needs met			
Bowel status assessed			
Patient satisfaction questionnaire completed			
Discharges only:			
TTOs ready			
Sick certificate obtained (if required) Form Med 3			
Complete **discharge checklist**			

Signatures, Name and Grade to be completed by Named Nurse for Shift			
	Signature	**Print Name**	**Print Grade**
Night Duty			
AM			
PM			
Night Duty			

Stage 4

Peterborough and Stamford Hospitals

NHS Foundation Trust

Cardiac Chest Pain/
Myocardial Infarction Pathway

*delete as appropriate

| Surname: |
| First Name: |
| Unit No. |
| Date of Birth: |
| Or patient label |

Date of discharge:
Diagnosis on discharge:

Discharge Plans	Signature/Print Name/Date
Discharge plans discussed with patient and family	
Exercise Test requested / MIBI Scan requested*	
Echocardiogram requested*	
Angiography referral sent + consent + "green card" given to patient	
Out-patient appointment requested Yes ☐ No ☐	
Anti-coagulation clinic* referral to commence/restart service	
Hospital transport home booked for: Date: Time:	
DNAR form copy for transport (see transport policy)	
Dr.'s discharge letter written (ensure **GTN** as TTO*)	
TTOs dispensed	
TTOs discussed with patient and/or family	
Sick certificate (if applicable) Form Med 3	
Other MDT advised of discharge date (document details below)	
All property returned to patient (including own medicines – PODs)	
Cardiac rehab & drug Information leaflets	
Cannula removed	
Patient satisfaction questionnaire completed	
Discharged on PAS	

Other requirements on discharge:

Date/Time	Progress Notes & Variances – reason and action taken	Signature/Name/Bp. No.

Index

i refers to an illustration; t refers to a table.

i refers to an illustration; t refers to a table.

i refers to an illustration; t refers to a table.

i refers to an illustration; t refers to a table.

i refers to an illustration; t refers to a table.